Leticia Preti Schleder

Spirituality in the face of illness

Leticia Preti Schleder

Spirituality in the face of illness

Spirituality of relatives of patients in an Intensive Care Unit

ScienciaScripts

Imprint

Any brand names and product names mentioned in this book are subject to trademark, brand or patent protection and are trademarks or registered trademarks of their respective holders. The use of brand names, product names, common names, trade names, product descriptions etc. even without a particular marking in this work is in no way to be construed to mean that such names may be regarded as unrestricted in respect of trademark and brand protection legislation and could thus be used by anyone.

Cover image: www.ingimage.com

This book is a translation from the original published under ISBN 978-613-9-66421-4.

Publisher:
Sciencia Scripts
is a trademark of
Dodo Books Indian Ocean Ltd. and OmniScriptum S.R.L publishing group

120 High Road, East Finchley, London, N2 9ED, United Kingdom
Str. Armeneasca 28/1, office 1, Chisinau MD-2012, Republic of Moldova, Europe
Printed at: see last page
ISBN: 978-620-8-02705-6

EPIGRAFE

LIFE TRAIN

"'A friend told me about a book that compared life to a train journey.

It's an extremely interesting comparison, when interpreted correctly. That's right, life is just a train journey, full of embarking and disembarking, some accidents, pleasant surprises on some journeys and great sadness on others.

When we are born, we get on this train and meet some people who, we think, will always be on this journey with us: Our parents.

Unfortunately, that's not true; at some point they'll come down and orphan us of their affection, friendship and irreplaceable company... But that doesn't stop interesting people, who will become very special to us, from getting on board during the journey.

Our brothers and sisters, friends and wonderful loved ones arrive. Many people take this train just for the ride, others will find only sadness on the journey, and still others will be on the train, ready to help those in need.

Many people get off and miss us forever, while others pass by in such a way that, when they get off, nobody even notices.

It's curious to realise that some passengers, who are so dear to us, sit in different carriages from us. So we have to travel separately from them. That doesn't stop us, of course, from crossing our carriage with great difficulty during the journey and reaching them...

But, unfortunately, we'll never be able to sit on it, because there will already be someone else occupying that seat. It doesn't matter, that's the journey, full of hitches, dreams, fantasies, waiting, goodbyes... But never returns.

So let's make this journey in the best possible way, trying to get on well with all the passengers. Looking for the best in each of them. Always remembering that, at some point during the journey, they may falter and we probably need to understand that. Because we too will often falter and there will certainly be someone who understands us.

The great mystery, after all, is that we'll never know which stop we're getting off at, let alone our companions, not even the one sitting next to us.

I wonder if, when I get off this train, I'll miss it....

I think I will. Parting with some of the friends I made on it will be painful, to say the least.

'Letting my children continue their journey alone will certainly be very sad. But I cling to the hope that, at some point, I'll be at the main station and I'll have the great thrill of seeing them arrive with luggage that they didn't have when they boarded...

And *what would make me happy would be to think that I had helped it grow and become valuable.*

Friends, let's make our stay on this train a peaceful one.

Let's make it worthwhile.

T, that when the time comes for us to disembark, our empty seat will bring nostalgia and good memories to those who continue the journey. "

Silvana Duboc

SUMMARY

Aim: to assess the Religious-Spiritual Coping (RSC) of family members of patients admitted to an intensive care unit (ICU). **Method:** a descriptive field study with a qualitative-quantitative approach. **Sample:** 45 relatives of ICU patients, 80% female and 20% male, aged between 18 and 65. **Data collection:** family members answered a questionnaire to characterise the sample and the CRE Scale. **Results:** the total CRE value in this study was 3.4 (expected value is between 1.00 and 5.00), which shows that the family members taking part in this study use CRE strategies. With regard to the CREN/CREP ratio, the value found was 0.7 (expected value ranges from 0.20 to 5.00), it was considered that the family members in this study make greater use of positive CRE strategies than negative ones. **Conclusions:** family members use positive ERC strategies more than negative ERC strategies during the process of hospitalising a family member in the ICU. This study also found that regardless of religion/spirituality, all family members believe in God and the majority believe that religion/spirituality has helped them to cope with the stress of hospitalisation.

Keywords: Spirituality, Psychological stress, Intensive care unit.

CHAPTER 1

INTRODUCTION

The motivation to carry out this research arose this year when I visited some of my university internships, and one place in particular caught my attention - the Intensive Care Unit (ICU) - because it is a place that has all kinds of technological devices, highly complex and invasive procedures and its beds are occupied by patients who are mostly in a "serious condition". This type of unit generates fear in the family member, "fear of the unknown", of the equipment, of the procedures, it causes anguish because they can't be with their family member 24 hours a day and doubt because they don't know if the patient will leave this place alive, thus generating stress due to hospitalisation.

During some of the family visits to the ICU, I realised that religion/spirituality was always present as a way of coping with this time of hospitalisation, whether through gestures, actions, words or religious accessories (rosary, bible), however, some doubts arose: is this type of coping positive or negative? In other words, do these family members use religion/spirituality as a form of support to get through the hospitalisation process or do they blame it for what is happening? With this in mind, we decided to carry out this research in order to identify the religious-spiritual *coping* strategies (RSCC) of these family members in order to assess the extent to which they use or blame their faith to cope with the stress of hospitalisation of a close relative.

The applicability of this research is valid, so that by identifying the *coping* strategies of these family members, the nursing team can start to develop nursing care focused on spiritual care, aiming for religion/spirituality as an ally in the treatment of the patient and in the insertion of the family member into the world of the ICU.

The spiritual dimension will form a new social paradigm. It is increasingly recognised that faith helps in the process of recovering health and coping with illness (SELLI and ALVES, 2007).

CHAPTER 2

LITERATURE REVIEW

2.1 *Coping* and Stress

There is no Portuguese translation of the word *Coping,* although many authors use the word enfrentamento as a synonym (KRISTENSEN, SCHAEFER and BUSNELLO, 2010).

Coping is conceived as a set of strategies used by people to adapt to adverse or stressful circumstances (ANTONIAZZI, DELL'AGLIO and BANDEIRA, 1998).

Coping is a set of cognitive and behavioural strategies used by individuals to manage stressful life situations (PANZINI and BANDEIRA, 2007).

Coping is a key concept that helps to understand adaptation and maladjustments in adaptation, since stress alone does not cause suffering and dysfunction (PANZINI, 2004).

Habitual ways of dealing with stress develop into *coping* styles, *which* can influence reactions in new situations and the extent of selected strategies (PANZINI and BANDEIRA, 2007).

There are *"coping* styles*"* and *"coping* strategies*",* and although the former can influence the latter, they are independent phenomena and have different theoretical origins. *Coping* styles refer to personality characteristics, i.e. the habitual ways a person uses to deal with perceived stress. The term *coping* strategies, on the other hand, refers to behaviours or cognitive actions taken in the course of a particular episode of stress, i.e. *coping* strategies are related to situational factors and can change from moment to moment during the stages of the stressful situation (ANTONIAZZI, DELL'AGLIO and BANDEIRA, 1998).

Since *coping* is a situational rather than dispositional process, indicating that there are no universal adaptive responses suitable for all individuals, in all situations and at all times, according to the situational perspective, *coping* is seen as a cognitive process that changes depending on the time and stress situation in which the individual is involved (DELL'AGLIO and HUTZ, 2002).

A stress response is any response involving a spontaneous emotional or behavioural reaction. The *coping* goal is the intention of a *coping* response, usually orientated towards reducing stress. There is a difference between coping outcomes, which are the specific consequences of the *coping* response, and stress outcomes, i.e. the immediate consequences of the stress response. Both may or may not promote the individual's adaptation (ANTONIAZZI, DELL'AGLIO and BANDEIRA, 1988).

The term "stress" has its meaning, popularly attributed to negative and deleterious effects on health. Some associate its occurrence with external factors, such as family and social responsibilities or the trials and tribulations of everyday life. Others define stress as the unpleasant physical sensations triggered by the adversities and challenges imposed by day-to-day life (TALARICO, 2009).

Stress develops when the tensions of everyday life prove to be greater than the individual's ability to master and/or overcome them, making it impossible for them to resist or create strategies to deal with them. Stress alters a person's quality of life, causing a decrease in the motivation needed for daily activities, especially in the challenges they encounter on a daily basis. It also causes a feeling of incompetence, with a consequent drop in self-esteem (LIPP and NOVAES, 2000).

Stress has also been defined as both a stimulus and a response. But a stimulus is only defined as stressful in terms of a stress response. The concept of stress emphasises the interaction between the person and the environment, taking into account the psychological characteristics of the person and the nature of the environmental event. It is parallel to the modern medical concept of illness, which understands that whether or not illness occurs also depends on the susceptibility of the individual's organism and not just on the action of an external organism on it (PANZINI, 2004).

Stress is associated with various changes in the functioning of the organism, including alterations both in physical systems (such as the endocrine system, immune system and nervous system) and in behavioural, emotional and cognitive systems. Many of these changes end up aggravating the individual's maladjustment to the developmental environment (GAZZANIGA and HEATHERTON, 2005).

It is not only the stimulus or the physical environment that determines the physiological response to stress, but the individual's evaluation of this stimulus and of themselves (TALARICO, 2005).

Associated with prolonged stress, the literature records the occurrence of organic diseases such as asthma, acne, skin problems (such as psoriasis and eczema), dysmenorrhoea, heart irregularities, hypertension, colitis, tumour formation, gastric ulcers, colds, herpes, mononucleosis, allergies and warts (PANZINI, 2004).

When people turn to religion to deal with stress, religious *coping* takes place, defined as the use of religious beliefs and behaviours to facilitate problem-solving and prevent or alleviate the negative emotional consequences of stressful life circumstances (KOENIG,

PARGAMENT and NIELSEN, 1988).

ORE describes how individuals use their faith to cope with stress and has been shown to be effective, with good rates of quality of life and physical and mental health. ORE strategies have been found to be particularly effective in the face of crisis situations, such as health problems, ageing, illness, disability, death, loss of loved ones and war (ZANCANARO, 2006).

CRE strategies can be categorised as positive or negative, depending on the consequences they have for those who use them.

Positive Religious-Spiritual *Coping* (CREP) is defined as encompassing strategies that provide a beneficial/positive effect for the practitioner, such as seeking love/protection from God or a greater connection with transcendental forces, seeking help/comfort in religious literature, seeking to forgive and be forgiven, praying for the well-being of others, solving problems in collaboration with God, redefining the stressor as beneficial, etc (PANZINI and BANDEIRA, 2007).

Negative Religious-Spiritual *Coping* (CREN) is defined as involving strategies that generate harmful/negative consequences for the individual, such as questioning the existence, love or actions of God, delegating the resolution of problems to God, feeling dissatisfaction/discontent in relation to God or members of a religious institution, redefining the stressor as divine punishment or evil forces, etc (PANZINI and BANDEIRA, 2007).

We can emphasise that those who use more CRE have a better physical, environmental, total and general quality of life, but especially a better psychological quality of life and social relationships (PANZINI, 2004).

2.2 Spirituality and Religion

Some people use the term spirituality as a synonym for religion, but these are two different concepts that differ from each other.

Spirituality has been dealt with on the basis of conceptual attributes determined for it, since there is no consensus on a globally accepted definition. In a way, the difficulty in assigning a scientifically acceptable concept stems, among other factors, from the difficulties in measuring and validating terminology that describes the phenomenon of Spirituality in its most original extension: that which is intimately related to an immaterial plane (PENHA, 2008).

Spirituality refers especially to a question of a personal nature: a response to fundamental aspects of life, a relationship with the sacred or the transcendent, which may (or may not) lead to the development of religious rituals and the formation of communities (SIQUEIRA, 2008).

Spirituality means that we are spiritual beings and temporarily possess a physical body (SELLI and ALVES, 2007).

To have and nurture spirituality, you don't need to profess a creed or belong to a religious institution. Spirituality is found in every person and at every stage of life, it is not the monopoly of a few, it is an integral part of the human constitution. It is therefore a universal human heritage (SANTA ROSA JÚNIOR, 2009).

The essence of spirituality is not to extirpate the evil that has plagued man, but to provide resources so that he can discover himself as the main person responsible for his own constructions (PENHA, 2008).

Although spirituality is closely linked to religion and the psychosocial dimension of the human being, it is different and unique. However, what makes it unique is not well understood (BENKO and SILVA, 1996).

We believe that man's spirituality is not only related to specific moments in his life (for example, the moment of death), but involves a personal positioning and reflection on the meaning of life itself (BENKO and SILVA, 1996).

Spirituality is an important aspect for those who experience a serious illness in the ICU or are close to death, as it helps them to cope with and accept pain and suffering by giving them some meaning. Regardless of the religious belief professed, a good relationship with God or a higher power allows the patient to understand and accept human suffering (SILVA, ARAÚJO and PUGGINA, 2009).

Spirituality is a personal feeling that stimulates an interest in others and in oneself, a sense of meaning in life that is able to withstand debilitating feelings of guilt, anger and anxiety (SAAD, MASIERO and BATTISTELLA, 2001).

Spirituality raises questions about the meaning of life and the reason for living, and is not limited to certain types of beliefs or practices. Religion is defined as the belief in the existence of a supernatural power, creator and controller of the universe, which has given man a spiritual nature that continues to exist after the death of his body. Religiosity is the extent to which an individual believes in, follows and practises a religion. Although there is considerable overlap between the notions of spirituality and religiosity, the latter differs from the other by clearly suggesting a specific system of worship and doctrine that is shared with a group. Personal beliefs can be any beliefs or values that an individual holds and which form the basis of their lifestyle and behaviour (FLECK et al, 2003).

Religion is a belief in the supernatural or in a divine force that has power over the universe and commands worship and obedience, a comprehensive code of ethics and philosophy; spirituality is a broader quality than religion. A person does not have to belong to an organised religion to achieve the spiritual (BENKO and SILVA, 1996).

Religiosity and spirituality are strongly rooted in a personal quest to understand life, its meaning and its relationship with the sacred or the transcendent. Thus, spiritual and/or religious beliefs and practices can address this need to seek a broader meaning to life and influence the way people interpret and deal with traumatic events (PERES and ALMEIDA, 2007).

Spirituality is often confused with religiosity, and the beliefs of others are not always understood, respected and accepted. Added to this is the fact that in the hospital context, and especially in the ICU, care for the biological body is prioritised to the detriment of care for the individual as a bio-psycho-spiritual being (SILVA, ARAÚJO and PUGGINA, 2009).

The need for religion/spirituality can come from verbal sources such as mass, worship, temples, shrines or from non-verbal sources, the so-called religious ornaments such as rosaries, the Bible, the Koran, etc.

Religious ornaments (rosaries, saints, pamphlets, bibles) are therefore non-verbal sources that indicate possible spiritual/religious needs because they convey faith and should be valued by professionals, since they predict the religious importance of the patient or family (PENHA, 2008).

A committed religious leader participates effectively in the construction of coping mechanisms. What's more, an effective religious leader also understands that the emotional and psychological pain of the sick person and their family can be eased or worsened by their attitude (SANTA ROSA JÚNIOR, 2009).

Since time immemorial, spiritual beliefs, practices and experiences have been one of the most prevalent and influential components of most societies. Health professionals, researchers and the general population have increasingly recognised the importance of the religious/spiritual dimension to health (ALMEIDA, 2009).

Spirituality remains important to the lives of the absolute majority of the world's population and it has been shown that religious involvement is generally related to better indicators of mental health and well-being (ALMEIDA, 2009).

Undoubtedly, the process of reclaiming the human values of care associated with the cultural importance of religious aspects as itinerants in the process of curing/rehabilitating illnesses have been fundamental mechanisms for bringing the discourse of Spirituality into health care (PENHA, 2008).

Much evidence indicates that patients experience less psychological stress when they re-establish a good relationship with God (or any other expression of the sacred) at critical moments of their illness, when they ask for forgiveness and when they manage to forgive their enemies, finding support, comfort and support (SILVA, ARAÚJO and PUGGINA, 2009).

The opportune moment for exercising our interiority is the time of illness! When we come face to face with the reality of the brevity of life here and realise how fragile our physical body is, then we wake up to the demands of the faculties and higher-order needs of our total being (which is not just matter). We are urged to admit our spirituality and awakened to see beyond the veil, beyond the physical plane and appearances (SANTA ROSA JÚNIOR, 2009).

Bioethics and spirituality are tools to help overcome the curative idea of health and turn to the empowerment of the individual, seen in its multiple dimensions (SELLI and ALVES, 2007).

Transferring responsibility to God can cause the patient and family a certain amount of anguish, given that at this time of life, belief systems can be in conflict and any indication of religion or false hope can directly interfere with coping with the illness (PENHA, 2008).

One factor that hinders spiritual care is the influence of materialism, which over-values beauty, power and material things, thus emptying human beings of the value they have in themselves as unique, intelligent, free, responsible and worthy beings (SELLI and ALVES, 2007).

The belief in a personal God and in the surrounding spiritual reality is transcendent, it is a primary truth, because it has such logical priority that it must be taken as admitted in order to make any observation or reflection possible; not that it is impossible to deny these truths, but that the mind is constrained by its very constitution to recognise them. No matter how hard man tries, he cannot banish this idea from his mind. These fundamental ideas cannot be subdivided or provoked by others. They are taken for granted in the acquisition of all knowledge. Therefore, their source lies in the cognitive power of the mind (SANTA ROSA JÚNIOR, 2009).

Spirituality or the spiritual path refers not only to the restructuring of the religious field itself, but also to fields such as psychology and medicine, in a movement in which new meanings, authorities and competences are in the process of being legitimised (SIQUEIRA, 2008).

2.3 Intensive Care Unit

ICUs are complex units for the care of critically ill patients, which require specific physical space, specialised human resources and advanced technological instruments, making them high-cost units (CIAMPONE et al, 2005).

ICUs arose from the need to improve environmental conditions, material resources and human resources with the technical, scientific and human capacity to care for critically ill, recoverable patients. This environment must provide conditions for observation, care and ongoing medical assistance. Considered an ideal place to provide care for acute patients with body dysfunctions who can benefit from this technological and human environment for health recovery, at the same time it can be seen and interpreted as highly stressful, cold, aggressive and traumatising for patients and their families (BETTINELLI and ERDMANN, 2009).

The technological apparatus of the ICU can impose fear and anguish on the patient and their family. The movement of people and the environment with the noise of this equipment can contribute to increased stress, fear and suffering for the patient and their family when they enter the ICU environment (BETTINELLI and ERDMANN, 2009).

In Brazil, the first ICUs were set up in the 1970s with the aim of centralising critically ill recoverable patients in a hospital area with human resources, equipment and materials specifically aimed at caring for these patients (KIMURA, KOIZUMI and MARTINS, 1997).

ICUs are important resources for the treatment of critically ill or potentially critically ill patients who require continuous and specialised care as a result of a wide variety of pathophysiological alterations. Treatment for these patients is provided by a specialised care team, in an environment where technological resources and sophisticated procedures can provide the conditions for reversing the patient's life-threatening disorders (KIMURA, KOIZUMI and MARTINS, 1997).

The need for technology to meet the expectations of life in the modern world is undeniable. However, the detriment of humanising characteristics in ICUs is an undeniable fact, since the focus of attention is directed towards procedures and the handling of increasingly precise devices of inestimable operational complexity, resulting in care that is often reduced to a few "bits" of buttons and volumes of medication (PENHA, 2008).

When thinking about care in the intensive care unit, it is important to emphasise that the health professions contemplate it as a discourse and a practice that, coherently or not, culminate in a multiplicity of manifestations. Each of these professions uses their knowledge of the world and their specific knowledge to provide this care (PINHO and SANTOS, 2008).

The ICU is an environment considered by many authors, professionals and patients to be stressful. This assessment can be understood as a result of the high level of movement of people, the sound of equipment, caring for serious, high-risk patients, intercurrences, living with situations of death and suffering, and the use of complex technologies that sometimes the workers themselves are not prepared to experience (STUMM et al, 2009).

Because it is a special environment, where severity, invasion and the risk of death are frequent, it seems that a stereotype is created that the ICU is a hostile, negative environment that produces little health, with the imagery of death, pain and suffering predominating (PINHO and SANTOS, 2008).

The ICU environment is a stressful factor for patients, staff and families, and is characterised by a climate of apprehension, a fast-paced routine, situations of imminent death, the use of advanced technological equipment with sound and light alarms (URIZZI, 2005).

There was also the recognition that the intensive care environment can, due to the characteristics of working with critically ill patients and their families, the use of technology and human relations, be a stress factor that adds to the problems of daily life outside the hospital to generate imbalance and possibly illness due to stress (DEZORZI and CROSSETTI, 2008).

The management of healthcare resources in an ICU is complex. It aims to recover the life and health of critically ill patients when possible. However, although it has the same objective, it must never lose sight of the human perspective and knowledge of the socio-cultural environment to which the sick person belongs (ALBÍSTUR et al, 2000).

The ICU environment, the physical layout, the systematisation of care and the established routines are usually detrimental to preserving the privacy and intimacy of patients and their families (BETTINELLI and ERDMANN, 2009).

In view of other research carried out using different methodological approaches, the Intensive Care Centre (ICU) is perceived by the family in a paradoxical way: at the same time as it inspires safety, due to the possibilities of therapeutic resources available, it frightens because of the strangeness of the place (URIZZI, 2005).

The diversity of ways in which families experience the hospitalisation of a family member can reveal important facets that make it possible to rethink the humanisation of care in its political, managerial and interpersonal dimensions, understanding that they are interrelated and need a process of reconstruction (URIZZI, 2005).

A significant point that emerges is the importance of the relationship established between the healthcare team and the family. Communication is fundamental, involving understanding the family's experience and being open to providing clear information, even if it is considered trivial. In other words, familiarity with the world of the ICU can lead the team to overlook how strange and even frightening the scenario is for the family (URIZZI, 2005).

Considering that hospitalisation in the ICU is something imposed on the family and felt with impact, familiarisation with this new reality occurs slowly and gradually (URIZZI, 2005).

In recent years, there has been a concern to introduce changes in ICUs in order to make the environment more welcoming and less impersonal. This humanisation process aims to change not only the physical space, but also the behaviour and attitudes of staff, patients and their families (FREITAS, 2005).

Humanising ICU care means integrating responsibility, sensitivity, ethics and solidarity with technical and scientific knowledge in caring for patients and their families and in interacting with the team. It involves relieving the pain and suffering of others; compassion, i.e. empathy translated into concrete solidarity; respect for the dignity and autonomy of others; understanding the meaning of life in its ethical, cultural, economic, social and educational aspects; and valuing the patient's human dimension over their pathology (SILVA, ARAÚJO and PUGGINA, 2009).

Since the ICU is a cold, mechanistic social space in which the imaginary is complex and at the same time ambivalent, making one rule more flexible would mean bringing distant families closer together, rather than keeping them apart, in order to allow the patients' state of health to recover along with their interpersonal bonds (PINHO and SANTOS, 2008).

The need for family members to be included in the ICU environment must be overcome in order to break the stereotype of a cold, "unknown" place that causes fear, anguish and stress, and to reinforce the need for humanisation in this unit; however, studies don't show us where this humanisation should take place. Much is said about understanding the meaning of the patient's and family member's life, respecting values and beliefs, but does the team interact with these values and beliefs? An example of this is the lingering doubt about the integration of care and spirituality in the world of intensive care (DEZORZI and CROSSETTI, 2008). In other words, we should talk about holistic care, encompassing all aspects, religion/spirituality, culture, social, educational, etc.

2.4 Family and the intensive care environment

The family is an institution that exerts a significant influence throughout the individual's development process and is generally seen as a group with a complex organisation that is inserted into a wider social context, maintaining constant interaction with it (BIASOLI-ALVES, 2004).

This is because the family, as a social group, also goes through a life cycle, which is dynamic and consists of certain stages, marked by both predictable critical events (marriage, children's adolescence) and unpredictable critical events (illness, loss). These events have a major impact on the family context, causing a crisis that directly or indirectly affects all its members (SUDBRACK, 2001).

Illness is an event that causes inconvenience not only for the patient, but also for their family members. Hospitalisation, when necessary, is seen as a crisis situation and generally represents a threatening experience that can compromise the balance of family dynamics to varying degrees (FREITAS, 2005).

Illness causes a lot of upheaval for the family. Tensions mount, everyone is completely focused on the drama of the illness and the many activities of daily life that had to be carried out normally are suddenly postponed, forgotten or even left behind. The home is then completely disorganised (SANTA ROSA JÚNIOR, 2009).

The breakdown of the family unit caused by illness and hospitalisation leads to an imbalance in the family's ability to function, generating conflicts, distancing and change (PETTENGILL and ANGELO, 2005).

The hospitalisation of a family member in the ICU usually occurs acutely and inadvertently, leaving little time for family adjustment. Faced with this stressful situation, family members may feel disorganised, helpless and unable to mobilise, causing different types of needs to emerge (FREITAS, 2005).

The process of hospitalisation can be considered a stressful but unique event for the patients and accompanying family members. In the case of the ICU admission process, a series of signs and symptoms of physical and emotional destabilisation can emerge. There are many factors that can cause this to happen, including temporary isolation, the risk to life, uncertainty about treatment and recovery, the imaginary surrounding the success and failure of attempts, as well as limitations in the provision of psychosocial support (GALA, TELLES and SILVA, 2003).

Hospitalisation in the ICU is identified as being more intense for family members than for patients, because it is experienced as a process of permanent adaptations, uncertainties and changes that affect the family's life history (URIZZI, 2005).

The patient's hospitalisation in the ICU is often a very difficult time for the family, who can experience feelings of uncertainty about their relative's present and future, feelings that also involve their own outlook on life (SILVA, ARAÚJO and PUGGINA, 2009).

In the family's experience, the threat to autonomy is identified from the illness situation and the conflicts that are established within the family itself. In this case, vulnerability is a human existential condition, due to the potential risk of injury perceived in the situation and which challenges the family's integrity (PETTENGILL and ANGELO, 2005).

When the patient is hospitalised, a life of responsibilities and activities is interrupted, and maintaining these is a clearly perceived concern for the family. Most of the time, everything is new and frightening for the family. There is no doubt that they need support, adequate information and to be close to the patient (SILVA, ARAÚJO and PUGGINA, 2009).

The greater the distance between the imaginary and reality, the greater the emotional stress for patients and their families (ALBÍSTUR et al, 2000).

That's why it's fundamental in intensive care to understand the family as an extension of the patient (PENHA, 2008).

It is believed that the patient is a segment of the visitors and that these are vitally important for the recovery of the person hospitalised in the ICU. These visitors need to be cared for by the nursing team in order to better manage the hospitalisation of the loved one in the ICU (SILVA DE SOUZA, CHAVES e SILVA, 2006).

We understand that the common sense that permeates the social imaginary of carers raises an interesting question about the complexity that the process of being admitted to the ICU represents for them, mixing the feeling of grief at the proximity of death with the negative view created by the amount of equipment that keeps patients alive in the unit (PINHO and SANTOS, 2008).

Family members often feel frustrated at not being with and caring for the patient, and guilty, out of a desire to make up for possible lost opportunities in the past. When anger, resentment and guilt present themselves in a phase of preparatory grief, the more the family can vent their grief, the better they will be able to bear the pain. The more the healthcare team can help relatives to vent their emotions, the more comforted they will feel (FREITAS,2005).

For some professionals, the lack of involvement with carers is due to a lack of time to devote fully to them, and the use of visiting hours as a time to hand them over so that their family member can look after them, keep an eye on them and be attentive (PINHO and SANTOS, 2008).

In general, people believe that the ICU environment is synonymous with imminent death for all patients and that intensive care professionals should have the concern, caution, responsibility and ethical commitment to educate patients and families, trying to change this meaning, adding greater value to care and providing support and guidance to the family, reducing their suffering at this time of ICU hospitalisation (BETTINELLI and ERDMANN, 2009).

Caring for the families of ICU patients allows them to build bonds during hospitalisation, enabling them to cope with moments of anguish and highly stressful suffering, as well as problems related to the repercussions of this event on the family's daily life. It is believed that families generally have the strength to cope; however, it is also up to intensive care professionals to make this explicit and, whenever necessary, to stimulate the emergence of new strengths (BETTINELLI and ERDMANN, 2009).

The process of separation, and perhaps the prospect of losing a loved one, is a multifaceted phenomenon that spreads throughout the family. Therefore, everyone's need to adapt is imperative, i.e. the shared recognition of reality, the common experience of loss and family reorganisation (BETTINELLI and ERDMANN, 2009).

It is believed that the peculiar characteristics of ICUs, especially in relation to the public or private nature of the institution to which they are linked, can generate specific needs in patients' families (FREITAS, 2005).

What the authors advocate is the need to include the family in the ICU environment in order to break down the "preconceptions" that are formed about them, improving care for the family and the patient.

In the day-to-day life of the ICU, the healthcare team spends more time developing their technical skills (hard technology) and cognitive skills (soft-hard technology) and little time using relationship technologies, such as welcoming the patient and even less time with the family (MARTINS et al, 2008).

Welcoming human anxieties and suffering can help re-signify ICU work and the hospitalisation process, minimising the conditions of mental suffering. The discourse that characterises care as a dimension that includes doing for the other, attentive listening and the inclusion of the family as an extension of the patients' social relationships seems to characterise the intention to organise practices around the logic of user-centred care, and not only on the illness or the immediate needs of the patients (PINHO and SANTOS, 2008).

Adequate, honest and uniform information is vital to avoid and reduce stress factors for both the patient and the family (MARTINS et al, 2008).

CHAPTER 3

OBJECTIVE

- To assess the Religious-Spiritual Coping of family members of patients admitted to an Intensive Care Unit.

CHAPTER 4

HYPOTHESIS

- Family members use a greater number of positive than negative coping strategies for stressful situations, i.e. they use religion/spirituality as an ally in managing the stress of hospitalisation.

CHAPTER 5

METHOD

5.1 Type of study

This is a descriptive field study with a qualitative and quantitative approach.

5.2 Using the instrument

The Religious-Spiritual *Coping* Scale (CRE Scale), adapted and validated for Brazilian culture (Anexol), was used to collect data. Factor analyses, internal consistency and correlation indicated that the CRE Scale is valid and reliable, evaluating positive and negative aspects of the use of religion/spirituality for stress management and constituting a comprehensive instrument, theoretically and empirically based, functionally orientated, clinically significant and useful for various areas of scientific research (PANZINI, 2004).

This instrument aims to assess the extent to which people turn to religion to deal with the stress of a family member's hospitalisation in an ICU. In order to achieve this goal, we focused the use of the scale on this specific situation, which may or may not be stressful. To do this, we replaced the phrase "Right now, think about the most stressful situation you have experienced in the last three years. Please describe it in a few words", with the phrase "Right now, think about the stress you are experiencing in this situation of a family member being hospitalised in an Intensive Care Unit.

CRE strategies can be divided into positive CRE and negative CRE strategies. The instrument contains 87 items in total, 66 positive and 21 negative.

The positive CRE contains 66 items divided into 8 factors, as follows: Transformation of Self and/or Life (P1), Actions in Search of Spiritual Help (P2), Offering Help to Others (P3), Positive Positioning Towards God (P4), Personal Search for Spiritual Growth (P5), Actions in Search of the Institutional Other (P6), Personal Search for Spiritual Knowledge (P7) and Distancing Through God, Religion and/or Spirituality (P8).

The negative CRE offered a 4-factor solution containing a total of 21 Items, called. Negative Reappraisal of God (N1), Negative Positioning towards God (N2), Negative Reappraisal of Meaning (N3) and Dissatisfaction with the Institutional Other (N4).

ERC scales can be useful in research and clinical practice, helping to deepen knowledge in the area or guiding the planning and implementation of appropriate interventions in health treatment contexts (PANZINI and BANDEIRA, 2007).

The CRE Scale presents questions with answers varying in 5 Likert-type ranges: "not at all", "a little", "more or less", "quite a lot" and "very much".

Firstly, the scale's internal consistency is assessed using Cronbach's alpha and then, in order to assess the participant using this scale, the value of positive CRE, negative CRE, the CREN/CREP ratio and the total CRE are computed.

5.3 Study site

The study was carried out in two hospitals, one in the interior of São Paulo, in the city of Jundiaí, the São Vicente de Paulo Charity Hospital (HCSVP) and the other at the SEPACO Hospital (Social Service of the Paper, Cardboard and Cork Industry of the State of São Paulo). Data was collected from the relatives of patients admitted to the ICUs.

- The HCSPV has three ICUs: a cardiac ICU with 8 beds, a general ICU with 16 beds and a neurological ICU with 6 beds.
- Sepaco has only one general ICU with 40 beds, distributed between surgical, clinical and palliative care, with the main demand being coronary patients and their complications.

5.4 Population

Family members of patients admitted to the HCSVP and Sepaco ICUs. The sample consisted of 45 research subjects, 28 relatives from HCSVP and 17 from Sepaco.

5.4.1 Inclusion Criteria

- Family members, first or second degree relatives of patients admitted to the ICU at the study site.
- Adult family members aged £18 and ^65.
- Family members of patients between the 5th° and 30th day of hospitalisation, i.e. at the critical moment of stress and change. We chose this period because we believe that there may be a period afterwards when the family adapts to the new situation and before that a difficult and confusing period when the situation is very new.

5.4.2 Exclusion Criteria

- Family members of patients admitted to hospital units other than the ICU.
- Elderly family members aged >65 years because of the possibility of cognitive

difficulties in answering the study questions.

- Family members of patients admitted to the ICU outside the period chosen for the study.

5.5 Data collection procedures

Initially, the work was sent to the Research Ethics Committee of the Jundiaí Medical School (FMJ) for approval, then authorisation was requested from the HCSVP ICU Coordination, where I explained what my research was about and how the data collection should take place, and I provided a copy of my project for the coordination to assess the proposal. After the HCSVP authorised the research, data collection began. At the Sepaco Hospital, a copy of the Sisnep cover sheet and the approval of the FMJ Ethics Committee were given to the Director in charge of the ICU, and once the research had been authorised, data collection began at this institution.

Family members of patients admitted to the general, cardiac and neurological ICUs at HCSVP and the general ICU at Sepaco were interviewed.

The family members were told about the research and its aims, which were to assess their religious-spiritual *coping* with the process of hospitalisation of a close relative. The family members were asked to read the Free and Informed Consent Form (FICF) (APPENDICES 1) with the researcher in order to answer any questions that arose. Two copies of the FICF were handed over, one to the researcher and the other to the family member.

Firstly, the family members answered the General Questionnaire to characterise the research subjects (Appendix 2) and then they answered the CRE Scale, where the appropriate response form was explained; this process took around 40 minutes to complete.

Puggina (2006) emphasises the importance of collecting data after the family member has visited the patient, so as not to cause any anxiety before the visit, such as the thought of bad news or a worsening clinical condition. However, the HCSVP coordinators authorised me to collect data only before the relatives' visits, during the wait for the visit and always accompanied by a psychology professional. The scale was filled in by the relatives and returned the same day.

At the Sepaco Hospital, data collection took place before the start of the visit. Family members were taken to a private room, where the purpose of the research was explained and the ICF and instrument were handed out and returned at the end of the visit. As the family members did not adhere to this form of data collection, and because it caused them some apprehension, it was discarded.

In an attempt to reach family members without causing any bad feelings, we carried out a new data collection, now during visiting hours, so we went from bed to bed, explaining the purpose of the research and handing out the ICF and the Instrument, to be returned at the end of the visit, but this only happened the next day, however, with greater participation from these family members.

CHAPTER 6

Data processing

The data was previously stored in *Microsoft Oficce Excel* for *Windows Explorer* and the quantitative data was analysed in the SAS (Statistical Analysis System) software version 9.01 by an expert[1] . The significance level was 5% and the software used for analysis was SAS version 9.1

Statistical analysis included characterising the sample in relation to the data from the general questionnaire using absolute (n) and relative (%) frequencies, and evaluating the psychometric parameters of the CRE Scale using the standard deviation, median, mean, maximum and minimum.The arithmetic mean is equal to the sum of all the values divided by the number of participants, while the median is the distribution point above and below which 50% of the cases lie (POLIT, BECK and HUNGLER, 2004).The standard deviation is the most widely used index of variability and represents the average deviation from the arithmetic mean, i.e. how much the scores varied on average from the arithmetic mean (POLIT, BECK and HUNGLER, 2004).

In order to better visualise the distribution of continuous data, it is convenient to establish ranges or intervals of variation, called classes. A class interval is defined as the extension of a class, which can be the difference between the two extreme values belonging to it, and which are called the lower and upper limits of the class. The number of classes depends on three factors: the total number of the sample, the total amplitude of the data (difference between the last and first values of the data sorted in ascending order, i.e. the largest minus the smallest) and the number of significant figures of the variable in which the data is expressed (ARANGO, 2001).In all the Tables with continuous data, the amplitude of the classes was established using the following method (VIEIRA, 2003):

- The number of classes should be approximately equal to the square root of the sample size:

$$\text{Number of classes} = \text{"V}n$$

---

[1] Sirlei Siani Moraes
Specialised in Statistics at the University of Campinas (UNICAMP)

CHAPTER 7

Results and Discussion

7.1 Sample characterisation

The sample consisted of 45 relatives of ICU patients, 28 relatives from HCSVP and 17 from Sepaco.

The 45 family members who took part in the survey were on average 37.5 years old (± 13.7 standard deviation), with a minimum age of 18 and a maximum of 64. Table 1 shows the distribution of the number of family members by age.

Table 1 - Distribution of family members according to age. Jundiaí, 2010.

Age	Number	Percentage
18-24	10	22,22%
24-30	4	8,88%
30-36	9	20%
36-42	7	15,55%
42-48	5	11,11%
48-54	2	4,44%
54-64	8	17,77%
Total	**45**	**100%**

The ages of the relatives varied greatly, but the majority were between 18 and 24 years old (10 of the 45; 22.22%). It is said that the advanced age of hospitalised relatives, as well as that of their spouses, who may also have health problems, can prevent them from accompanying their partners during hospitalisation, which contributes to the greater frequency of children on visits, which justifies the prevalence of young people on ICU visits in the study (Lautert, Echere Unicovsky, 1998).The sample was made up predominantly of females (36 of the 45; 80%) and only 9 of the 45 (20%) of males (Graph 1).

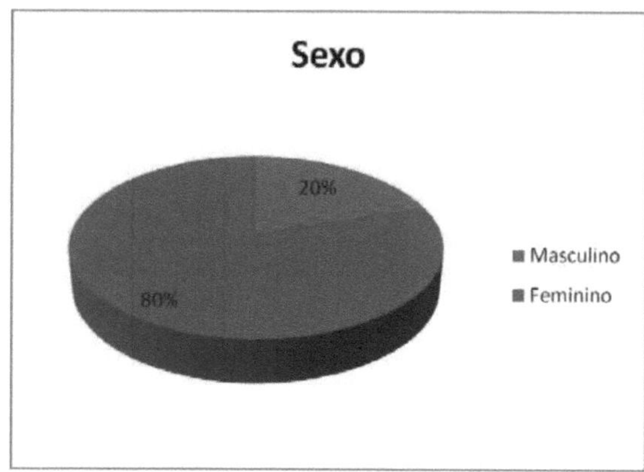

Graph 1- Distribution of family members according to gender. Jundiaí, 2010.

This fact becomes concrete in this group of carers, since the presence of women with patients is intended to meet some of the needs of these individuals, mainly from the point of view of safety, providing emotional support in a moment of crisis, or ultimately caring for the patient. This role has been played by women since the dawn of humanity (LAUTERT, ECHER and UNICOVSKY, 1998).

It seems to us that in moments of crisis, as is the case with illness, and where there is a need for a carer, it is the family, and especially the woman, who ends up playing this role (LAUTERT, ECHER and UNICOVSKY, 1998).

In terms of level of education, most of the interviewees (36 per cent) had completed high school, which may make it easier for family members to understand the information provided (ALMEIDA et al, 2009) (Graph 2).

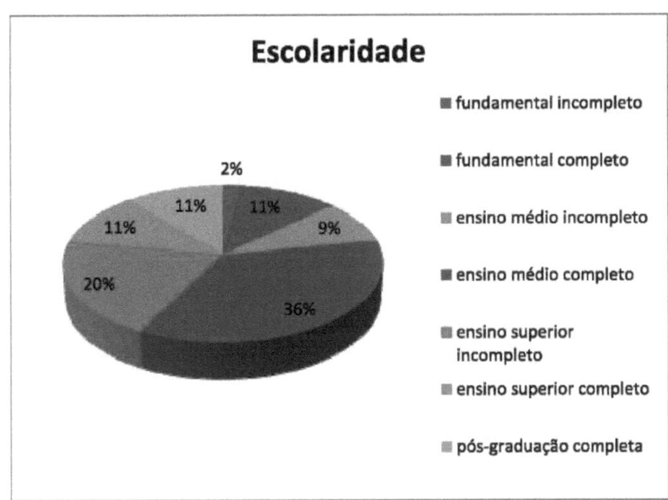

Graph 2- Distribution of family members according to schooling. Jundiaí, 2010.

A high level of schooling can be considered a positive factor, since reading and writing presupposes a certain level of understanding, which can improve the results of research and guidance (Lautert, Echer and Unicovsky, 1998).With regard to monthly income, the majority of family members earn up to 5 minimum wages (17 out of 45; 38 per cent), which is to be expected, given that the data was collected in public hospitals (Graph 3).

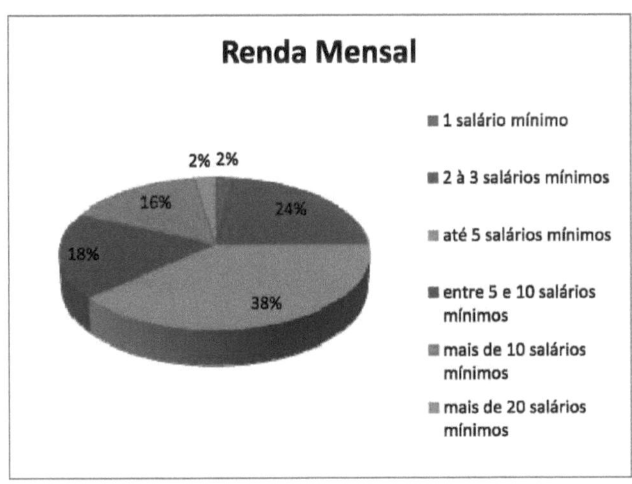

Graph 3 - Distribution of family members according to monthly income. Jundiaí, 2010.

As for the family members' marital status, the majority were married, 21 out of 45 (47 per cent), 16 (36 per cent) were single and the rest were divorced, 5 (11 per cent), widowed, 1 (2 per cent) and 2 (4 per cent) other (Graph 4).

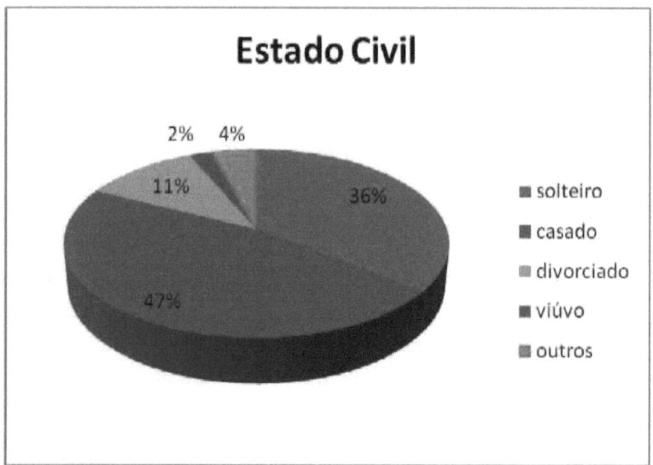

Graph 4 - Distribution of family members according to marital status. Jundiaí, 2010.

When asked if they believed in God, the answer was unanimous: 100 per cent believed in God.

Despite not having concrete proof of God's existence, culture, religion and the scriptures (Bible) lead us to believe in the existence of this Being, whether through the letters written by the prophets that speak of his existence, the miracles performed by Jesus as a work of God and even the creation of the world as a service of God, which makes us believe in his existence.

With regard to how long they had believed in God, 41 of the 45 family members (91 per cent) had always believed, 3 (7 per cent) had believed for more than 10 years and 1 (2 per cent) had believed for more than 5 years (Graph 5).

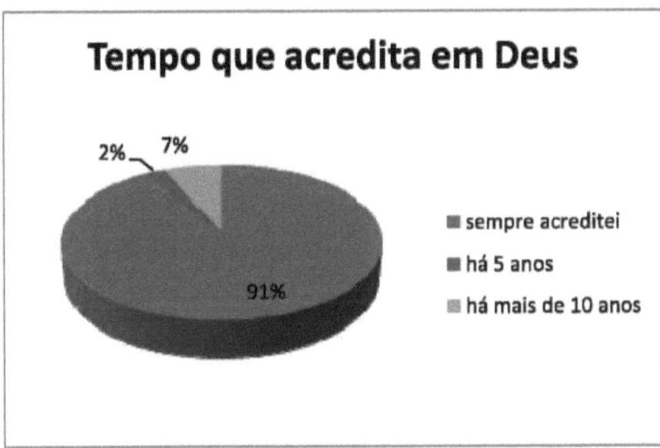

Graph 5- Distribution of family members according to how long they have believed in God. Jundiaí, 2010.

The family plays an important role in preserving and changing habits, customs and behaviours among its members and between generations (SUÁREZ and GALERA, 2004).

And although the majority of familymembers have always believed in God, because we were introduced to a religion by our family as children and came to believe in this God, some family members have only recently come to believe in God, which we can justify by the socialising process, because it is through this process that the individual develops their identity, acquiring the values, beliefs, models and ideas necessary for their social performance (ROMANELLI, 2002).

With regard to religion, 29 of the 45 family members (65%) were Catholic, 9 (20%) had no specific religion but considered themselves spiritualised, 5 (11%) were evangelical, 1 (2%) atheist and 1 (2%) Umbandist (Graph 6).

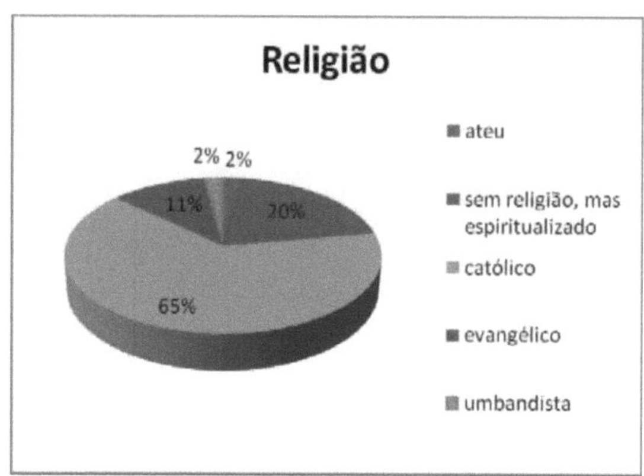

Graph 6- Distribution of family members according to their religion. Jundiaí, 2010.

Brazil is a country of great religious diversity. For the purposes of comparison with the sample in this research, we can point to data from the Demographic Census (Instituto Brasileiro de Geografia e Estatística/IBGE, 2000), which indicates the percentage of the Brazilian resident population by declared religion: Roman Catholic 73.6%, Evangelicals 15.4%, Spiritists 1.3%, No religion 7.4%, Umbanda 0.3% and other religions 1.8%. These percentages shown in the Census are proportional to those found in this research.

Spirituality is what gives meaning to life and is a broader concept than religion, which is an expression of spirituality (SAAD, MASIERO and BATTISTELLA, 2001). Spirituality is more related to the reason for living without necessarily containing a belief and religion is related to beliefs in a supernatural power.

A Catholic is someone who follows the doctrine of Catholicism.

An Evangelical is a person who follows the principles of the Gospel and belongs to non-Catholic religious groups (MICHAELIS, 2000).

An atheist who does not believe in the existence of God (MICHAELIS, 2000).

Umbanda is a religious cult that combines Afro-Brazilian elements with spiritism (MICHAELIS, 2000).

Spiritism is the doctrine according to which the spirits of the dead communicate with the living, mainly through the action of mediums (MICHAELIS, 2000).

Individuals without religion, but who are spiritualised, are based on the existence of the soul and of God (MICHAELIS, 2000).

With regard to changing religion, 36 of the 45 family members (80%) have never changed their religion and 9 (20%) report that they have already changed their religion (Graph 7).

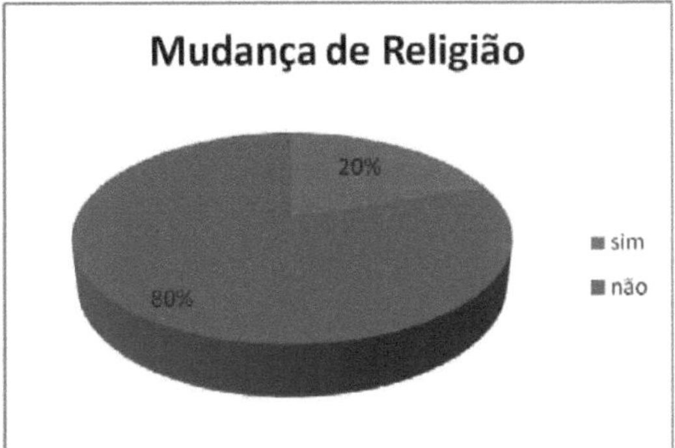

Graph 7 - Distribution of family members according to change of religion. Jundiaí, 2010.

This change of religion can happen because people are introduced to religions by their family members very early on, and as they grow up and difficulties arise, people change religions in search of the one they identify with most. When asked about the importance of religion/spirituality in the event of stress in any circumstance, 19 of the 45 family members (43%) thought religion was important, 13 (29%) thought it was very important, 11 (24%) relatively important, 1 (2%) somewhat important and 1 (2%) didn't think it was important (Graph 8).

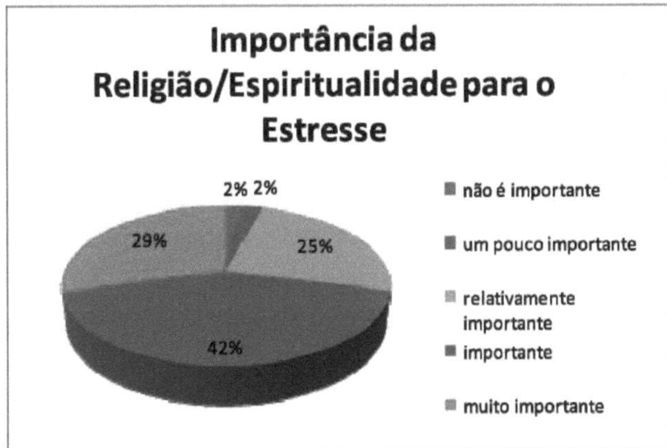

Graph 8 - Distribution of family members according to the importance of religion/spirituality in dealing with stress. Jundiaí, 2010.

It is important to emphasise that in addition to religion/spirituality, family members can choose other sources to deal with this stressful time, such as social isolation, medical help or psychological help.

Regarding the importance of religion in their lives, 31 (69 per cent) family members said it was very important, 5 (11 per cent) not important, 5 (11 per cent) important, 3 (7 per cent) relatively important and 1 (2 per cent) somewhat important (Graph 9).

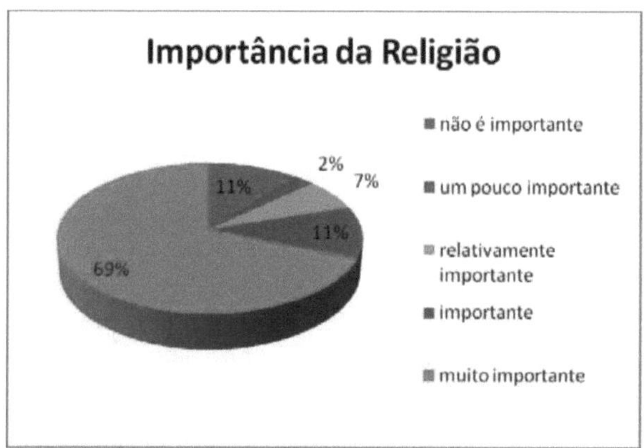

Graph 9- Distribution of family members according to the importance of religion for them. Jundiaí, 2010.

The importance of religion in people's lives may be related to the religion they follow, as each religion preaches a different doctrine. This high percentage of people who believe that religion is important in their lives alerts us to the importance of spiritual care in hospitals, both for patients and their families. Nurses need to be aware of and sensitive to these issues in order to provide appropriate care.

With regard to attendance at religious meetings, there was a variation in responses and small differences in numbers between them: 11 of the 45 family members (24 per cent) attend religious meetings once a week, 10 (22 per cent) twice a month, 8 (18 per cent) once a month, 7 (16 per cent) rarely, 5 (11 per cent) more than once a week and 4 (9 per cent) never (Graph 10).

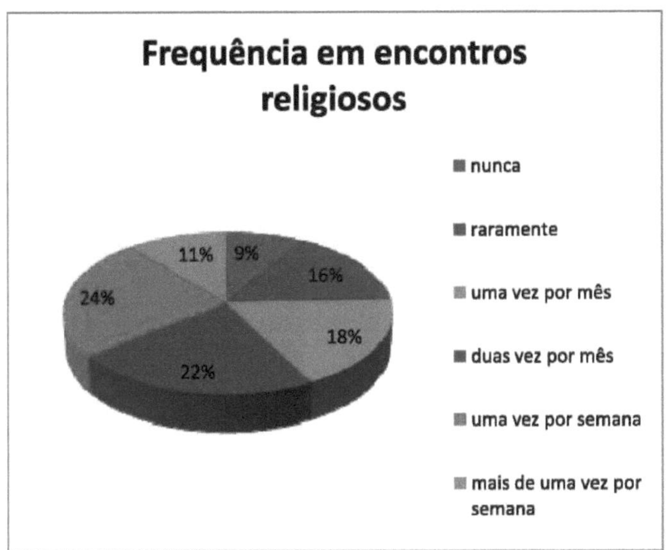

Graph 10- Distribution of family members according to their attendance at religious meetings. Jundiaí, 2010.

Attendance at religious meetings varies according to the religion of the family members and the importance and adoration they have for it. This also varies according to the religion followed, as each one preaches a different type of religious meeting, some varying from weekly to daily meetings. Some people use the artefact of a busy social life as an obstacle to attending more religious meetings.

When asked about the time dedicated to private religious activities, we can see two extremes of responses with minimal difference in percentage, 14 of the 45 family members (31 per cent) dedicate themselves to these activities more than once a day and 13 (29 per cent) rarely dedicate themselves, the rest divided into 8 (18 per cent) dedicate themselves once a day, 3 (7 per cent) two to three times a week, 3 (7 per cent) never, 2 (4 per cent) once a week and 2 (4 per cent) once a month (Graph 11).

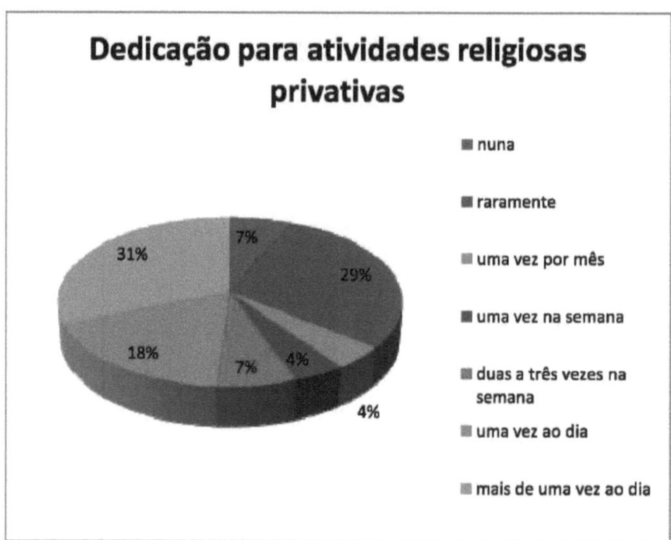

Graph 11- Distribution of family members according to their dedication to private religious activities. Jundiaí, 2010.

These differences in time devoted to religious activities can vary according to the fervour of each family member and the need they feel to practise these activities, which range from prayer, meditation, chanting and studying sacred books (Bible, Koran).

With regard to how much Religion/Spirituality has helped them cope with stress, 25 of the 45 family members (56%) say it has helped a lot, 15 (33%) say it has only helped, 3 (7%) have not helped, 1 (2%) has helped a little and 1 (2%) has helped more or less (Graph 12).

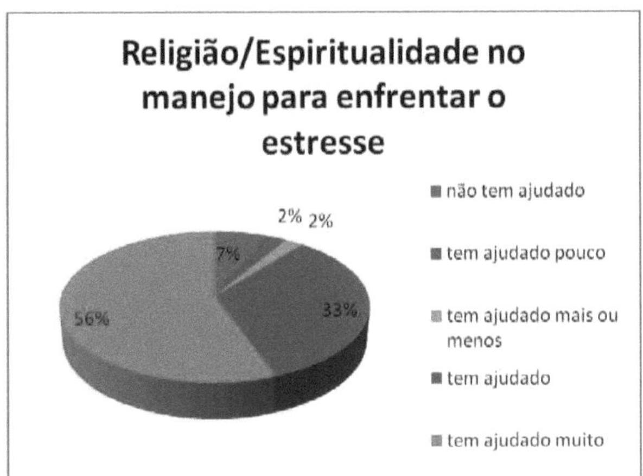

Graph 12 - Distribution of family members according to the use of their religion/spirituality in coping with stress. Jundiaí, 2010.

Family members (participants in the ICU care process) need attention, welcome and support, as they often don't know who to turn to in these moments of anguish and suffering. They are invariably susceptible to stress, as their daily lives undergo sudden changes as a result of this event (BETTINELLI and ERDMANN, 2009). It is at this point that they turn to religion/spirituality to deal with the stress, which is why most family members report that religion/spirituality has helped them a lot in managing stress.

The questions below were used to identify the changes related to spirituality that family members have been undergoing as a result of the stressful event they are going through, in this case the hospitalisation of a family member in the ICU.Regarding the spiritual growth of family members, 20 of the 45 (44%) reported that it has been growing, 10 (22%) it has been growing a little, 8 (18%) it has been growing a lot, 4 (9%) it has been growing more or less and 3 (7%) it has not been growing (Graph 13).

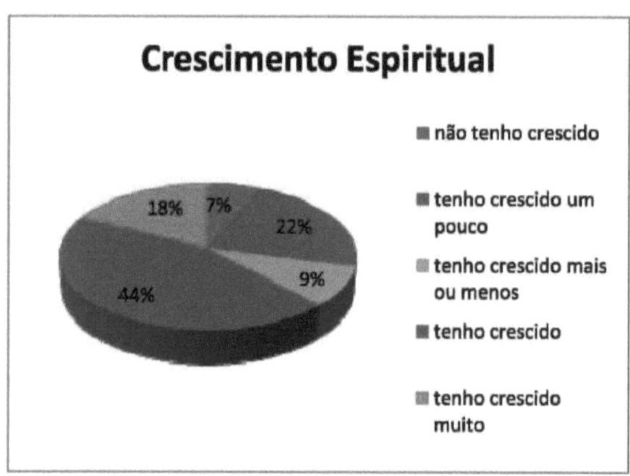

Graph 13 - Distribution of family members according to their spiritual growth - Jundiaí, 2010.

The majority of family members, 20 out of 45 (44%), report that they have grown spiritually during this stressful time of hospitalisation. We can justify this by the fact that at this time they are fragile and some seek religion/spirituality to get through this time, which leads them to this spiritual growth.In terms of growth with God, 20 of the 45 family members (45%) report that they have grown a lot, 10 (22%) have grown, 7 (16%) have grown more or less, 6 (13%) have grown a little and 2 (4%) have not grown (Graph 14).

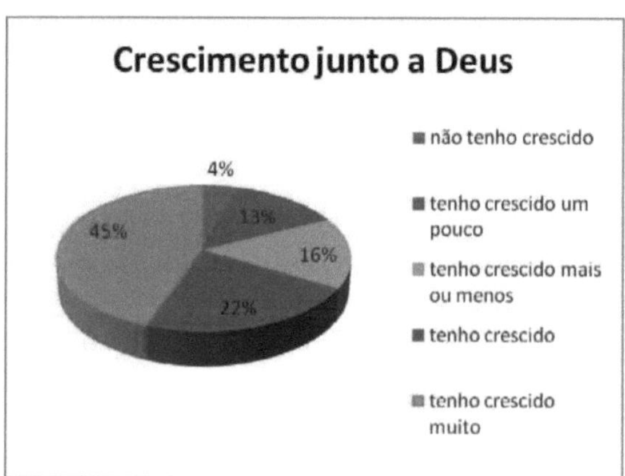

Graph 14- Distribution of family members according to their growth with God. Jundiaí, 2010.

Although most family members feel that they have grown a lot with God, this varies according to the religion they follow, as some religions don't even believe in the existence of God. In terms of spiritual growth with the religious institution, 14 of the 45 family members

(31 per cent) have grown, 12 (27 per cent) have not grown, 9 (20 per cent) have grown a little, 6 (13 per cent) have grown more or less and 4 (9 per cent) have grown a lot (Graph 15).

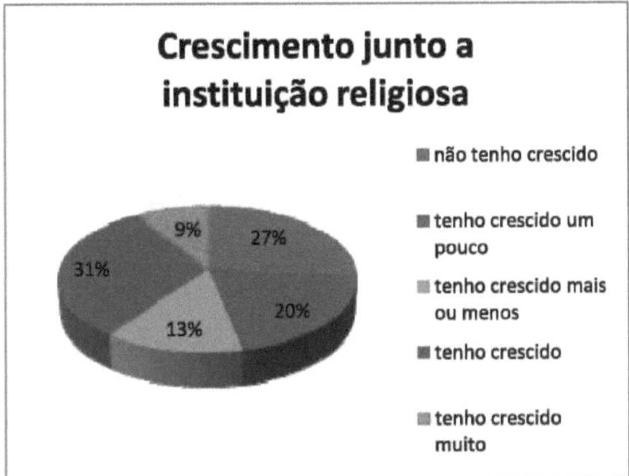

Graph 15- Distribution of family members according to their growth with the religious institution. Jundiaí, 2010.

When asked about their growth with their religious institution, there was little difference between one answer and the next, and although most family members feel they have grown with their religious institution, some don't feel its support, which leads them to believe that they haven't grown or that they have grown little.

Regarding the classification of family members' health, 24 of the 45 (53 per cent) considered it good, 14 (31 per cent) very good, 4 (9 per cent) poor and 3 (7 per cent) neither bad nor good (Graph 16).

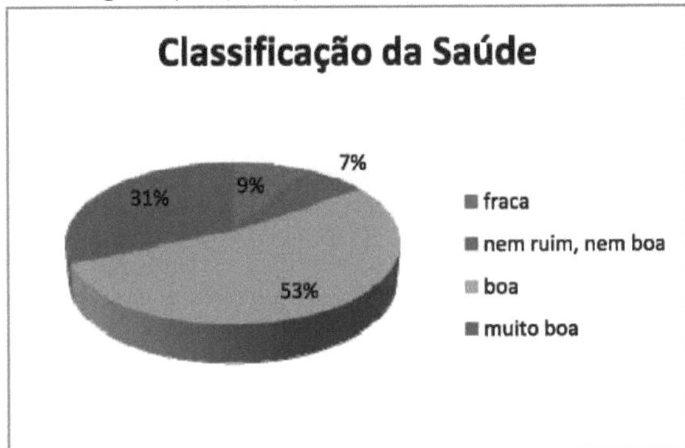

Graph 16- Distribution of family members according to their health classification.Jundiaí, 2010.

Although most of the family members taking part in this survey were aged between 18 and 24, they rated their health as good, which could be explained by the fact that nowadays health problems range from illnesses to incapacitating accidents. Since the middle of the 20th century, with the change in the epidemiological profile of a large part of the population, epidemiological studies have also started to focus on other types of diseases, illnesses and events, such as non-infectious diseases (cancer, diseases of the circulatory system, diseases of the respiratory system, for example), illnesses and injuries resulting from external causes (traffic accidents, illnesses and accidents at work, homicides, poisonings, etc.), nutritional disorders (nutritional deficiencies, etc.).), nutritional disorders (malnutrition, anaemia, obesity, etc.) and risk factors for illness or death (smoking, hypercholesterolaemia, low birth weight, etc.) (SOARES, ANDRADE, CAMPOS, ANO).

With regard to the health status of family members, the vast majority, 40 out of 45 (89%), consider themselves healthy and only 5 (11%) consider themselves ill (Graph 17).

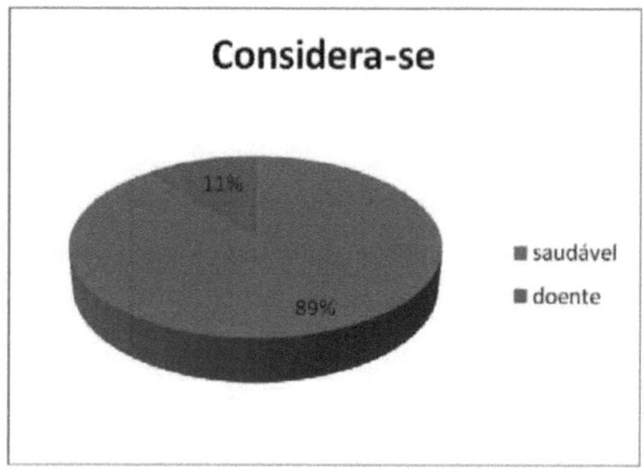

Graph 17- Distribution of family members according to their health condition. Jundiaí, 2010.

This may be related to the fact that most of the family members taking part in this survey are aged between 18 and 24. As for health problems, 31 of the 45 family members (69 per cent) reported having no health problems and 14 (31 per cent) reported having health problems (Graph 18).

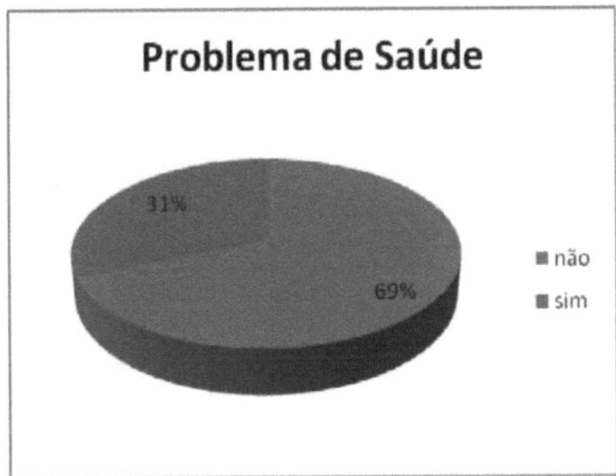

Graph 18- Distribution of family members according to health problem. Jundiaí, 2010.

The vast majority reported having no health problems and this may be related to lifestyle, healthy eating habits, physical activity and even the age of the family members interviewed.

7.2 Religious-Spiritual Coping Scale

Firstly, the CRE Scale was assessed for internal consistency using Cronbach's Alpha and then for values using the mean, standard deviation, median, minimum and maximum.

L. J. Cronbach published an almost encyclopaedic article in 1951 in which he discussed the problems associated with estimating the internal consistency of a scale or test and other authors' proposals for calculating it. In this article, Cronbach considers the previous derivations and, assuming no limits in the classification pattern of the items, formalises a proposal for estimating internal consistency based on the variances of the items and the test totals per subject, which became known as Cronbach's "alpha" index (MAROCO and MARQUES, 2006).

Cronbach's alpha is a useful tool for investigating the reliability of a measure and therefore allows the accuracy of an instrument to be studied (MAROC and MARQUES, 2006).

Generally speaking, the lower the variability of intra-subject responses and the higher the variability of inter-subject responses, the higher the Alpha. On the other hand, Alpha is generally higher when there is homogeneity of inter-item variances than when there is not (MAROCO and MARQUES, 2006).

The scale had an excellent internal consistency index of 0.923, which can be up to 1 and must be higher than 0.70. With regard to the positive items, an index of 0.942 was obtained, considered high, and each of the domains had values close to and with the same meaning (positive) as the coefficient found (Table 2).

Table 2- Cronbach's Alpha internal consistency indices - positive CRE

Measure	Value
Cronbach's Alpha Coefficient - Positive	0,942
Transforming yourself and/or your life	0,930
Actions in search of spiritual help	0,935
Offering help to others	0,930
Positive attitude towards God	0,938
Personal Search for Spiritual Growth	0,934
Actions in search of the institutional other	0,931
Personal search for spiritual knowledge	0,944
Detachment through God, religion and/or spirituality	0,934
Cronbach's Alpha Coefficient - Total	**0,923**

The operational definitions of the eight factors of the Positive CRE Dimension of the CRE Scale are described below.

FACTOR P1: TRANSFORMATION OF YOURSELF AND/OR YOUR LIFE - Any CRE behaviour that results in a personal transformation, be it an internal change in the person practising it and/or an external change in their life.

P2 FACTOR: ACTIONS IN SEARCH OF SPIRITUAL HELP - All CRE behaviour in which the person makes a move to seek some kind of spiritual help from others, whether individual, institutional, family or social.

FACTOR P3: OFFERING HELP TO OTHERS - All CRE behaviour in which the person seeks to help others, whether individual, institutional, family or social.

P4 FACTOR: POSITIVE POSITIONING TO GOD - All CRE behaviour that exposes a personal positioning towards God in relation to the situation. It can be manifested through CRE styles, setting religious boundaries, seeking support in God.

FACTOR P5: PERSONAL SEEK FOR SPIRITUAL GROWTH - All CRE behaviour that reveals either an individual search for God and/or spirituality (as opposed to an institutional search), or a search for oneself through God and/or spirituality.

FACTOR P6: ACTIONS IN SEARCH OF THE INSTITUTIONAL OTHER - All CRE behaviour that moves closer to the institutional. In other words, a rapprochement with the locals, members or religious representatives.

FACTOR P7: PERSONAL SEEK FOR SPIRITUAL KNOWLEDGE - All CRE behaviour in which the person seeks greater religious-spiritual knowledge.

FACTOR P8: GETTING AWAY FROM GOD, RELIGION AND/OR SPIRITUALITY - Change in personal perspective on the situation, in which the person gets away from the problem by getting closer to God and/or religious/spiritual issues. In other words, any CRE behaviour that someone performs in order to get closer to God, religion or spirituality.

With regard to the representation of negative items, the index was slightly lower at 0.732, although acceptable, and each of the domains showed values with the same sign (negative) and close to the coefficient found (Table 3).

Table 3- Cronbach's Alpha internal consistency indices - CRE Negative

Measure	Value
Cronbach's Alpha coefficient - Negative	0,732
Negative Reappraisal of God	0,767
Negative stance towards God	0,609
Negative Reappraisal of Meaning	0,564
Dissatisfaction with the other Institutional	0,719
Cronbach's Alpha Coefficient - Total	**0,923**

Below is the definition of the four factors of the Negative CRE Dimension of the CRE Scale:

FACTOR N1: NEGATIVE RE-EVALUATION OF GOD - Any CRE behaviour that constitutes a negative cognitive re-evaluation of the person's idea of God, whether of his characteristics, behaviour, etc., raising questions about this God and his designs.

FACTOR N2: NEGATIVE POSITIONING IN FRONT OF GOD - All CRE behaviour in which the person asks or simply expects God to take control of the situation and be responsible for resolving it, without their individual participation

FACTOR N3: NEGATIVE REEVALUATION OF SIGNIFICANCE - Any ERC behaviour in which the person negatively re-evaluates the significance of the situation as an act and/or consequence of evil or as a punishment for their own actions, lifestyle, mistakes, sins, etc.

FACTOR N4: INSATISFACTION WITH THE INSTITUTIONAL OTHER - All CRE behaviour that reveals feelings of dissatisfaction, disgust or hurt with any institutional representative.

Therefore, according to the cronbach's alpha analysis, the questionnaire can be considered, in this sample, to have excellent internal consistency in general, for positives, and good internal consistency for negatives, with the CREP Dimension and its factors, for the most part, performing better than the CREN Dimension and its factors in terms of accuracy, as well as a greater number of items.

The total CRE had a mean of 3.4 ± 0.6, ranging from 2.6 to 4.1. The domains were described using mean, standard deviation, median, minimum values (lowest value in the sample) and maximum values (highest value in the sample) (Table 4).

Table 4 - Average values found in the sample for CRE

CRE	Averag	Standard Deviation	Median	Minimum	Maximum
Total CRE	3,4	0,3	3,4	2,6	4,1

Positive CRE	2,7	0,8	2,7	1,4	4,5
Negative CRE	1,9	0,6	1,7	1,1	3,4
CREN/CREP	0,7	0,2	0,7	0,4	1,4
Positive					
Transforming yourself and/or your life	3,0	1,0	3,1	1,3	4,8
Actions in Search of Spiritual Help	2,2	1,0	1,9	1,0	4,3
Offering Help to Others	2,5	1,1	2,4	1,0	4,6
Positive Positioning Towards God	3,5	0,6	3,7	1,9	4,3
Personal Search for Spiritual Growth	2,8	1,0	2,8	1,2	5,0
Actions in Search of the Institutional Other	2,4	1,1	2,1	1,0	5,0
Personal Search for Spiritual Knowledge	1,8	0,9	1,6	1,0	5,0
Away Through God, Religion and/or Spirituality	3,2	1,0	3,3	1,2	4,8
Negatives					
Negative Reappraisal of God	1,6	0,8	1,3	1,0	4,4
Negative stance towards God	2,7	0,9	2,8	1,3	5,0
Negative Reappraisal of Meaning	1,7	0,8	1,2	0,8	3,8
Dissatisfaction with the Institutional Other	1,5	0,5	1,3	1,0	3,0

To assess the participant using this scale, four main indices are considered: two dimensional and two general. The first two relate to each of the two dimensions of the CRE Scale. They are important for indicating the different types of CRE practised by the person being assessed, as well as their respective levels, and are the basic measures of this scale. The last two indices integrate all the information provided by the scale by relating the first two measures in order to obtain general indices using all the items on the CRE Scale. Thus, they point to the interaction between the basic measures, showing a profile of all the behaviours performed/evaluated (PANZINI, 2004).

The scores and domains were calculated according to the methodology proposed by the Brazilian validation of the questionnaire.

• **Positive CRE:** index obtained from the average of the 66 questions in the CREP dimension of the CRE Scale. Value between 1.00 and 5.00. The higher the score, the greater the use of positive religious-spiritual coping.

The average value obtained for positive CRE in this study was 2.7, which is within the expected range. With this average value, we can conclude that family members use CRE strategies habitually.

Among the averages achieved by the positive CRE factors, the one with the highest value was P4 "Positive attitude towards God", and the lowest was P7 "Personal search for spiritual knowledge". This same result was found in the study by Panzini (2004), which analysed the CRE Scale and its relationship with health and quality of life.

Therefore, we can conclude that the family members in this study, in relation to the situation of a family member's hospitalisation, make greater use of CREP styles, where religious boundaries are established, seeking support in God and a greater connection with him, and make less use of the search for greater religious-spiritual knowledge.

• **Negative CRE:** index obtained from the average of the 21 questions in the CREN dimension of the CRE Scale. Values are between 1.00 and 5.00. The higher the score, the greater the use of negative religious-spiritual coping.

With regard to the value of negative CRE, the result found was 1.9, and as this is considered a relatively low value, we conclude that family members use negative CRE strategies to a lesser extent.

In relation to the averages reached by the negative CRE factors, the one with the highest value was N2 "Negative position towards God" and the lowest was N4 "Dissatisfaction with the institutional other", the result of the lowest value was different to that found in the research by Panzini (2004) who presented N1 "Negative re-evaluation of God" as the factor with the lowest value.

Therefore, in terms of CREN strategies, the family members in this study hope that God will take control of the situation and that he will resolve it, their prayers intend to change God's will and the least used CREN strategy is the feeling of dissatisfaction with some institutional representative, be they a member, attendee or leader of the religious institution.

• **CREN/CREP ratio:** an index that shows the percentage of CREN used in relation to the total CREP, obtained by simply dividing them (CREN/CREP ratio = CREN/CREP). The value of the ratio can be between 0.20 and 5.00. The higher this value, the greater the use of CREN in relation to the use of CREP and the lower this value, the greater the use of CREP in relation to CREN; therefore, this index is inversely proportional, as the person is expected to have a higher positive CRE index in relation to the negative CRE index, due to the positive and negative consequences they entail, respectively.

In this study, the CREN/CREP ratio was 0.7, which was within the expected range, and because it was low, we believe that the family members in this study make greater use of positive CRE strategies than negative ones.

The ratio between CREP and CREN (ratio CREN/CREP=0.70) in this study indicates that, on average, the participants used 70 per cent CREN of the amount of CREP used, which is close to the ratio proposed by Panzini (2004) as being the minimum to obtain a final positive result: 2CREP: 1CREN (ratio CREN/CREP_<0.50). In this same study, Panzini showed a ratio of CREN/CREP=0.54, which is also within the parameters of the proposed ratio.

• **Total CRE:** index that shows the **total** amount of CRE practised by the person being evaluated. It is obtained from the average between the positive CRE index and the average of the inverted answers to the 21 negative CRE items in the CREN dimension (inverted CREN=average). Therefore, total CRE= Average [positive CRE, inverted negative CRE], a value between 1.00 and 5.00.

As for total ERC, since the two dimensions have opposite directions, its calculation is made possible by the inversion and the higher its value, the greater the total use of ERC by the person being assessed. Finally, to assess the extent to which the person uses certain ERC strategies, an index (P1 to P8/N1 to N4) was calculated for each factor, calculated as the average of the questions that make them up (PANZINI, 2004).

The values found for total ERC in this study ranged from a minimum of 2.6 to a maximum of 4.1, with an average of 3.4, which is within the expected range, and because it is considered to be a high value, it proves that the family members taking part in this study use ERC strategies in large numbers. In his study, Panzini (2004) found minimum values of 2.53 and maximum values of 4.76, with an average of 3.80, a result similar to that found in this study.

We can conclude from all these factors that the family members in this study use positive ERC strategies more than negative ERC strategies during the process of hospitalising a family member in the ICU.

CHAPTER 8

CONCLUSIONS

Most of the family members who took part in this survey were female, aged between 18 and 24, had completed high school, had a monthly income of up to 5 minimum wages and were married. With regard to religion, the majority declared themselves Catholics and had never changed their religion. They reported that religion was very important to them and said that they attended religious meetings once a week and rarely engaged in private religious activities.

This study also found that regardless of religion/spirituality, all family members believe in God and most believe that religion/spirituality has helped them a lot in coping with stress.

With regard to the changes they have identified in themselves during the process of hospitalisation of a family member, the majority said that they have grown spiritually and with the religious institution and that they have grown a lot with God. We can therefore conclude that religion/spirituality is intrinsically positively related to coping with stressful situations.

We therefore observed that family members use positive ERC strategies more than negative ERC strategies during the process of hospitalising a family member in the ICU.

Thus, the hypothesis raised in this study that family members use a greater number of positive CRE strategies than negative ones to cope with stressful processes, such as the hospitalisation of a family member, was proven through the average CREN/CREP ratio.

CHAPTER 9

FINAL CONSIDERATIONS

As psychologists are the only professionals legally authorised to administer psychological tests, the fields of Psychology of Religion and Coping are relatively new in our country. This creates difficulties, as there is still a long way to go in terms of theory and many barriers to overcome (PANZINI, 2004). Therefore, nursing professionals should pay attention to the subject of religion and *coping,* seeking to improve the quality of care and expand their technical and scientific knowledge of these uncovered issues.

The ERC strategies used can reveal the feelings of these patients and their families, which the healthcare team focused on providing care doesn't visualise, so that these feelings can interfere with the patient's recovery and the family member's illness, which can include depression, anxiety, stress, etc.

Therefore, by identifying these *coping* strategies of family members, the healthcare team can begin to think about strategies focussed on Spiritual Assistance, aiming for religion/spirituality as an ally in the treatment of the patient and in the insertion of the family member into the world of the ICU.

The reaction of family members when they were approached to take part in the survey was interesting, as some showed excitement, compared to others who showed a certain resistance. This was because the survey was about religion, a topic that everyone deals with in their own way, depending on the doctrine they follow, and also because it was a survey that sought out family members at a difficult time, such as the hospitalisation of a relative.

That's why there's a need for studies on Religion/Spirituality in order to end the taboo that people feel when talking about this subject.

LIMITATIONS OF THE STUDY

- It took some time for the HCSVP coordinators to authorise this research, as it involved relatives of ICU patients. The research was directed at the institution's psychologists and data collection could only take place when they were present, which made it difficult to collect data in time, as the demand came from these professionals.

- The physical space and the lack of a private location at the HCSVP made it impossible to collect the data after the visits, so the questionnaire was administered beforehand, which caused a certain amount of apprehension among family members, and because some were anxious and distressed about what they would find in the ICU, they preferred not to take part in the survey, reducing the number of participants.

- Family members found it difficult to understand some of the questions and terms in the CRE Scale and reported that the instrument was long and sometimes had repetitive questions.

- Because it's a complex instrument that requires attention and the location doesn't allow it, we can't guarantee that the family members understood all the questions and answered them accordingly.

REFERENCES

ALBÍSTUR, M.C.; et al. La familia del paciente internado en la Unidad de Cuidados Intensivos. **Rev Med Uruguay,** Uruguay, vol.16, pp.243-256, 2000.

ALMEIDA, A.M. Espiritualidade & Saúde Mental: O desafio de reconhecer e integrar a espiritualidade no cuidado com nossos pacientes. **Zen Review,** 2009.

ALMEIDA, A.S.; ARAGÃO, N.R.O.; MOURA, E.; LIMA, G. de C.; HORA, E.C.; SILVA, L.A.S.M. Sentimentos dos familiares em relação ao paciente internado na unidade de terapia intensiva. **Revista Brasileira de Enfermagem,** Brasília vol.62, n.6, Nov./Dec.2009.

ANTONIAZZI, A. S.; DELL'AGLIO, D. D.; BANDEIRA, D. R. The concept of coping: A theoretical review. **Estudos de Psicologia,** Natal, vol.3, n.2, pp.273-294,1998.

ARANGO, H.G. **Theoretical and computational biostatistics.** Rio de Janeiro: Guanabara Koogan, 2001.235p.

BENKO, M.A.; SILVA, M.J.P. da. Thinking about spirituality in undergraduate teaching. **Rev. Latino-Am. Enfermagem,** Ribeirão Preto, vol.4, n.1, pp.71-85, January 1996.

BETTINELLI, A.L.; ERDMANN, A.L. Hospitalisation in an Intensive Care Unit and the family: perspectives on care. **Avances en Enfermería,** vol. XXVII, n.1, pp. 15-21, jan./jun. 2009.

BIASOLI-ALVES, Z.M.M. Researching and intervening with families with diverse loved ones. In: ALTHOFF, C.R.; ELSEN, I.; NITSCHKE, R.G. (Orgs.). Florianópolis: Papa-livro Editora, 2004. pp.91-106.

CIAMPONE, J.T.; GONÇALVES, L.A.; MAIA, F.O.F.; PADILHA, K.G. Nursing care needs and therapeutic interventions in the Intensive Care Unit: a comparative study between elderly and non-elderly patients. **Acta Paulista de Enfermagem,** São Paulo, vol.19, n.1, pp. 28-35, 2006.

DELL'AGLIO, D.; HUTZ, C.S. Coping strategies of children and adolescents in stressful events with peers and adults. **Psicologia USP,** São Paulo, vol. 13, n.2, pp .203-225, 2002.

DEZORZI, L.W.; CROSSETTI, M.G.O. Spirituality in self-care for nursing professionals in intensive care. **Revista Latino-Americana Enfermagem,** Ribeirão Preto, vol.16, n.2, March/April 2008.

FLECK, M.P.A.; BORGES, Z.N.; BOLOGNESI, G.; ROCHA, N.S. Development of the WHOQOL, spirituality, religiosity and personal beliefs module. **Rev Saúde Pública,** vol.37, n.4, pp. 446-55, 2003.

FREITAS, K.S. Necessidades de familiares em Unidades de Terapia Intensiva: análise comparativa entre hospital público e privado.[dissertação]. São Paulo: **School of Nursing, University of São Paulo,** 2005.

GALA, M.F.; Telles, S.C.R.; Silva, M.J.P. Occurrence and meaning of touch among nursing professionals and patients in a surgical ICU and Semi-Intensive Unit. **Rev Escola de Enfermagem da USP,** vol.37, n.1, pp. 52-61,2003.

GAZZANIGA, M.S.; HEATHERTON, T.F. Psychological science: Mind, brain and behaviour. **Artes Médicas,** Porto Alegre, 2005.

Brazilian Institute of Geography and Statistics/IBGE. **Percentage distribution of the resident population by religion - Brazil - 1991/2000. Demographic Census 1991/2000.** Available at http://www.ibge.gov.br/7a12/conhecer brasil/defaultphp?id tema menu=2&id te ma submenu=5. Accessed on 4 November 2010.

KIMURA, M.; KOIZUMI, M.S.; MARTINS, L.M.M. Caracterização das unidades de terapia intensiva do Município de São Paulo. **Rev.Esc.Enf. USP, São Paulo,** vol.31, n.2, pp.304-315, August 1997.

KOENIG, H.G.; PARGAMENT, K.I.; NIELSEN, J. Religious coping and health status in medically ill hospitalised older adults. **The Journal of nervous and mental disease,** vol.186, n.9, pp. 513-521,1998.

KRISTENSEN, C.H.; SCHAEFER, L.S.; BUSNELLO, F. de B. Coping strategies and stress symptoms in adolescence. **Estudos de Psicologia,** Campinas, vol. 27, n.1, pp. 21-30, January/March 2010.

LAUTERT, L.; ECHER, I.C.; UNICOVSKY, M.A.R. O Acompanhante do paciente adulto hospitalizado. **Revista Gaucha de Enfermagem,** Porto Alegre, vol. 19, n.2, pp.118-131, July 1998.

LIPP, M.E.N.; NOVAES, L. O stress. São Paulo: Contexto, 2000.

MAROCO, J.; MARQUES, T.G. How reliable is cronbach's alpha? Old questions and modern solutions? **Instituto Superior de Psicologia Aplicada,** Portugal,Laboratório de

Psicologia vol.4, n.1, pp. 65-90, 2006.

MARTINS, J.J.; NASCIMENTO, E.R.P.; GEREMIAS, C.K.; SCHNEIDER, D.G.; SCHWEITZER, G.; MATTIOLI, H.N. Welcoming the family in the Intensive Care Unit: knowledge of a multiprofessional team. **Rev. Eletr. Enf.** [Internet], vol.10, n.4, pp.1091-101,2008.

MICHAELIS: **Minidicionário escolar da língua Portuguesa.** São Paulo, Companhia Melhoramentos, 2000.

PANZINI, R.G.; BANDEIRA, D.R. Religious-Spiritual Coping Scale (CRE scale): Elaboration and Validation of Construct. **Psicologia em Estudo,** Maringá, vol.10, n.3, pp.507-516, Sep./Dec. 2005. Available at:

http://www.scielo.br/scielo.php?script=sci_arttext&pid=S1413-73722005000300019&lng=en&nrm=iso. Accessed on 10 December 2009.

PANZINI, R.G.; BANDEIRA, D.R. Religious/spiritual coping. **Revista Psiquiátrica Clínica,** São Paulo, vol.34, supl.1, pp. 126-135, 2007.

PANZINI, R.G. Escala de Coping Religioso Espiritual (Escala CRE): Translation, Adaptation and Validation of the RCOPE Scale, Addressing Relations with Health and Quality of Life. 238f. Dissertation (Master's Degree in Psychology) - **Federal University of Rio Grande do Sul - Institute of Psychology** - R.G Sul, 2004.

PENHA, R.M. A expressão da dimensão espiritual no cuidado de enfermagem em UTI [dissertation]. São Paulo: **School of Nursing, University of São Paulo;** 2008.

PERES, J.; ALMEIDA, A.M. Restorative Spirituality. **Psique Ciência&Vida,** São Paulo, pp. 44-50, 2007.

PETTENGILL, M.A.M.; ANGELO, M. Vulnerability of the family: Development of the concept. **Rev Latino-am Enfermagem,** vol.13, n.6, pp.982-988, nov./dez. 2005.

PINHO, L.B.; SANTOS, S.M. The dialectic of humanised care in the ICU: contradictions between the discourse and the professional practice of nurses. **Revista Escola de Enfermagem da USP,** São Paulo, vol.42, n.1, pp.66-72, 2008.

POLIT, D.F.; BECK, C.T.; HUNGLER, B.P.; **Fundamentals of Nursing Research: methods, evaluation and utilisation.** 5ed. São Paulo: Artmed, 2004. 487p.

PUGGINA, A.C.G. The use of music and vocal stimuli in comatose patients: relationship between auditory stimuli, vital signs, facial expression and the Glasgow and Ramsay Scales. 157f. Dissertation (Master's in Nursing). **USP School of Nursing,** São Paulo, 2006.

ROMANELLI, G. Authority and power in the family. In: CARVALHO, M.C.B (Org.). **A família contemporânea em debate** (pp. 73-88). São Paulo: EDUC/Cortez, 2002.

SAAD, M.; MASIERO, D.; BATTISTELLA, L.R. Evidence-based spirituality. **Acta. Fisiátrica,** vol.8, n.3, pp.107-112, 2001.

SANTA ROSA JÚNIOR, H. Relationships of transpersonal care in the pastoral accompaniment of HIV-positive people: a case study [dissertation]. **School of Theology.**

São Leopoldo, 2009.

SELLI, L.; ALVES, J.S. O cuidado espiritual ao paciente terminal no exercício da enfermagem e a participação da bioética. **Centro Universitário São Camilo,** São Paulo, vol.1, n.1, pp.43-52, 2007.

SILVA DE SOUZA, S.R.O.; CHAVES, S.R.F.; SILVA, C.A. Visits in the ICU: an encounter between strangers. **Rev. Bras. Enferm.,** vol.59, n.5, pp. 609-13, Sep/Oct, 2006.

SIQUEIRA, D. The Western Religious Labyrinth. From Religion to Spirituality. From the Institutional to the Unconventional. **Sociedade e Estado,** Brasília, vol. 23, n.2, pp. 425-462, May/August, 2008.

SOARES, D.A.; ANDRADE, S.M. de; CAMPOS, J.J.B.de. Epidemiology and Health Indicators. **Bases of Collective Health.** Year

SUÁREZ, R.E.; GALERA, S.A.F. Discurso de los padres sobre el uso de drogas lícitas e ilícitas percibido por estudiantes universitários. **Revista Latino- americana de Enfermagem,** vol.12(especial), pp.406-411,2004.

SUDBRACK, M.F.O. Systemic family therapy. In: SEIBEL, S.D.; TOSCANO JÚNIOR, A. (Org.). **Dependência de drogas** (pp. 403-415). São Paulo: Ed. Atheneu, 20001.

SUTMM, E.M.F.; et al. Quality of life, stress and repercussions on care: nursing staff in an intensive care unit. **Revista Textos & Contextos,** Porto Alegre, vol.8, n.1, pp. 140-155, jan./jun., 2009.

TALARICO, J.N.S. Stress and coping in elderly people with Alzheimer's disease. Master's thesis. **School of Nursing, University of São Paulo.** São Paulo, 2005, 138f.

TALARICO, J.N.S. Stress, cortisol concentrations and coping strategies in memory performance of healthy elderly people with mild cognitive impairment and Alzheimer's disease [PhD]. **School of Nursing, USP,** 2009.

URIZZI, F. Experiences of relatives of patients in intensive care: the other side of hospitalisation. 139f. Dissertation (Master's in Nursing) - University of São Paulo - **Ribeirão Preto School of Nursing,** São Paulo, 2005.

VIEIRA, S. Elements of Statistics. 4ed. São Paulo: Atlas, 2003.168p.

ZANCANARO, L.G. Religious/Spiritual *Coping* in patients undergoing cancer treatment. 71 f. Monograph (Bachelor of Physiotherapy). **Assis Gurgacz College,** Cascavel, 2006.

ANNEX 1
CRE SCALE

Religious-Spiritual *Coping* Scale
PANZINI AND BANDEIRA (2005) - BRAZILIAN VERSION OF THE RCOPE SCALE (PARGAMENT, KOENIG & PEREZ, 2000)
DEVELOPED AT THE FEDERAL UNIVERSITY OF RIO GRANDE DO SUL
INSTITUTE OF PSYCHOLOGY - POSTGRADUATE COURSE IN DEVELOPMENTAL PSYCHOLOGY

We're interested in whether and how much you use religion and spirituality to deal with stress in your life. Stress happens when you realise that a certain situation is difficult or problematic because it goes beyond what you think you can bear, threatening your well-being. The situation may involve you, your family, your work, your friends or something that is important to you.

Right now, think about the stress you are experiencing in this situation of a family member being hospitalised in an intensive care unit.

The phrases below describe attitudes that can be taken in stressful situations. Circle the number that best represents **how much YOU did or didn't do what is written in each sentence to deal with the stressful situation** you described above.
As you read the sentences, understand the meaning of the word God according to your own belief system (what you believe).

Example:
I tried to make sense of the situation through God.
(1) not at all (2) a little (3) more or less (4) a lot (5) very much

If you **haven't** tried at **all** to make sense of the situation through God, circle the number (1)
If you've tried **a little,** circle (2)
If you've tried **more or less,** circle (3)
If you've tried **hard enough,** circle (4)
If you've tried **really hard,** circle (5)

Remember: There is no right or wrong option
Mark only one alternative in each question.
Be honest with your answers and don't leave any questions
blank!

1. I prayed for the well-being of others
(1) not at all (2) a little (3) more or less (4) a lot (5) a lot

2. I sought God's love and protection
(1) not at all (2) a little (3) more or less (4) a lot (5) a lot

3. I asked for God's help to forgive other people
(1) not at all (2) a little (3) more or less (4) a lot (5) a lot

4. I rebelled against God and his designs
(1) not at all (2) a little (3) more or less (4) a lot (5) a lot

5. I sought a greater connection with God
(1) not at all (2) a little (3) more or less (4) a lot (5) a lot

6. I questioned God's love for me
(1) not at all (2) a little (3) more or less (4) a lot (5) a lot

7. I didn't do much, I just waited for God to solve my problems for me
(1) not at all (2) a little (3) more or less (4) a lot (5) a lot

8. I went to a religious or prayer centre
(1) not at all (2) a little (3) more or less (4) a lot (5) a lot

9. I wondered if evil had anything to do with this situation
(1) not at all (2) a little (3) more or less (4) a lot (5) a lot

10. I tried to work for social welfare
(1) not at all (2) a little (3) more or less (4) a lot (5) a lot

11. I begged God to make everything work out
(1) not at all (2) a little (3) more or less (4) a lot (5) very much

12. I sought protection and guidance from spiritual entities (saints, spirits, orishas, etc.)
(1) not at all (2) a little (3) more or less (4) a lot (5) a lot

13. I looked to God for strength, support and guidance
(1) not at all (2) a little (3) more or less (4) a lot (5) a lot

14. I tried to get together with others who had the same faith as me
(1) not at all (2) a little (3) more or less (4) a lot (5) a lot

15. I felt dissatisfied with the religious representatives of my institution
(1) not at all (2) a little (3) more or less (4) a lot (5) a lot

16. I read books on spiritual/religious teachings to understand and deal with the situation
(1) not at all (2) a little (3) more or less (4) a lot (5) a lot

17. I asked God to help me find a new purpose in life
(1) not at all (2) a little (3) more or less (4) a lot (5) a lot

18. I struggled to receive comfort from my religious beliefs
(1) not at all (2) a little (3) more or less (4) a lot (5) a lot

19. I searched for love and care for the members of my religious institution
(1) not at all (2) a little (3) more or less (4) a lot (5) a lot

20. I tried to stop thinking about my problems, thinking about God
(1) not at all (2) a little (3) more or less (4) a lot (5) a lot

21. I went to a religious temple
(1) not at all (2) a little (3) more or less (4) a lot (5) a lot

22. I did the best I could and handed the situation over to God
(1) not at all (2) a little (3) more or less (4) a lot (5) a lot

23. I wondered if God was chastising me for my lack of faith
(1) not at all (2) a little (3) more or less (4) a lot (5) a lot

24. Practised acts of moral and/or material charity
(1) not at all (2) a little (3) more or less (4) a lot (5) a lot

25. I felt that God was working with me
(1) not at all (2) a little (3) more or less (4) a lot (5) a lot

26. I prayed to God that things would be all right
(1) not at all (2) a little (3) more or less (4) a lot (5) a lot

27. I thought about spiritual matters to divert my attention from my problems
(1) not at all (2) a little (3) more or less (4) a lot (5) very much

28. Through religion I understood why I was suffering and tried to change my behaviour to improve the situation
(1) not at all (2) a little (3) more or less (4) a lot (5) a lot

29. I sought advice from my higher spiritual guide (guardian angel, mentor, etc.)
(1) not at all (2) a little (3) more or less (4) a lot (5) very much

30. I turned to God to find a new direction in life
(1) not at all (2) a little (3) more or less (4) a lot (5) very much

31. I tried to provide spiritual comfort to other people
(1) not at all (2) a little (3) more or less (4) a lot (5) very much

32. I wondered if God had abandoned me
(1) not at all (2) a little (3) more or less (4) a lot (5) very much

33. I asked God to help me be better and make fewer mistakes
(1) not at all (2) a little (3) more or less (4) a lot (5) very much

34. I thought it might bring me closer to God
(1) not at all (2) a little (3) more or less (4) a lot (5) very much

35. I didn't try to deal with the situation, I just waited for God to take my worries away
(1) not at all (2) a little (3) more or less (4) a lot (5) very much

36. I felt that evil was trying to take me away from God
(1) not at all (2) a little (3) more or less (4) a lot (5) very much

37. I handed the situation over to God after doing everything I could
(1) not at all (2) a little (3) more or less (4) a lot (5) very much

38. I prayed to discover the purpose of my life
(1) not at all (2) a little (3) more or less (4) a lot (5) very much

39. I performed spiritual acts or rites (any action specifically related to your belief: sign of the cross, confession, fasting, purification rituals, quoting proverbs, chanting mantras, psychography, etc.) (1) not at all (2) a little (3) more or less (4) a lot (5) a lot

40. I acted in collaboration with God to solve my problems
(1) not at all (2) a little (3) more or less (4) a lot (5) a lot

41. I wondered if my religious institution had abandoned me
(1) not at all (2) a little (3) more or less (4) a lot (5) a lot

42. I focussed my thoughts on religion to stop worrying about my problems
(1) not at all (2) a little (3) more or less (4) a lot (5) a lot

43. I searched for a total spiritual reawakening
(1) not at all (2) a little (3) more or less (4) a lot (5) a lot

44. I sought spiritual support from the leaders of my religious community
(1) not at all (2) a little (3) more or less (4) a lot (5) a lot

45. I prayed for a miracle
(1) not at all (2) a little (3) more or less (4) a lot (5) a lot

46. Followed spiritual advice to improve myself physically or psychologically
(1) not at all (2) a little (3) more or less (4) a lot (5) a lot

47. I trusted that God was with me
(1) not at all (2) a little (3) more or less (4) a lot (5) a lot

48. I sought spiritual help to overcome my resentments and hurts
(1) not at all (2) a little (3) more or less (4) a lot (5) a lot

49. I sought God's mercy
(1) not at all (2) a little (3) more or less (4) a lot (5) a lot

50. I thought God didn't exist
(1) not at all (2) a little (3) more or less (4) a lot (5) a lot

51. I questioned whether even God has limits
(1) not at all (2) a little (3) more or less (4) a lot (5) a lot

52. Watched religious or spiritual programmes or films
(1) not at all (2) a little (3) more or less (4) a lot (5) a lot

53. I became convinced that evil forces were at work to make all this happen
(1) not at all (2) a little (3) more or less (4) a lot (5) a lot

54. I sought help or comfort in religious literature
(1) not at all (2) a little (3) more or less (4) a lot (5) a lot

55. I offered spiritual support to my family, friends...
(1) not at all (2) a little (3) more or less (4) a lot (5) a lot

56. I asked for forgiveness for my mistakes
(1) not at all (2) a little (3) more or less (4) a lot (5) a lot

57. I took part in spiritual healing sessions
(1) not at all (2) a little (3) more or less (4) a lot (5) a lot

58. I acted in partnership with God, collaborating with Him
(1) not at all (2) a little (3) more or less (4) a lot (5) a lot

59. I wondered if God had allowed this to happen to me because of my mistakes
(1) not at all (2) a little (3) more or less (4) a lot (5) a lot

60. Attended religious/spiritual services or sessions
(1) not at all (2) a little (3) more or less (4) a lot (5) a lot

61. I tried to do the best I could and let God do the rest
(1) not at all (2) a little (3) more or less (4) a lot (5) a lot

62. I voluntarily got involved in activities for the good of others
(1) not at all (2) a little (3) more or less (4) a lot (5) a lot

63. I listened to and/or sang religious songs
(1) not at all (2) a little (3) more or less (4) a lot (5) a lot

64. I knew I couldn't handle the situation, so I just waited for God to take over
(1) not at all (2) a little (3) more or less (4) a lot (5) a lot

65. I evaluated my actions, thoughts and feelings, trying to improve them
according to religious teachings
(1) not at all (2) a little (3) more or less (4) a lot (5) a lot

66. I received help through the laying on of hands (passes, prayers, blessings,
magnetism, reiki, etc.)
(1) not at all (2) a little (3) more or less (4) a lot (5) very much

67. I sought help through meditation
(1) not at all (2) a little (3) more or less (4) a lot (5) a lot

68. I've sought or had spiritual treatments
(1) not at all (2) a little (3) more or less (4) a lot (5) a lot

69. I tried to deal with the situation in my own way, without God's help
(1) not at all (2) a little (3) more or less (4) a lot (5) a lot

70. I tried to find a teaching from God in what happened
(1) not at all (2) a little (3) more or less (4) a lot (5) a lot

71. I tried to build a strong relationship with a higher power
(1) not at all (2) a little (3) more or less (4) a lot (5) a lot

72. I bought or subscribed to periodicals that talked about God and spiritual
matters
(1) not at all (2) a little (3) more or less (4) a lot (5) very much

73. I felt that my religious group seemed to be rejecting or ignoring me
(1) not at all (2) a little (3) more or less (4) a lot (5) very much

74. Participated in religious or spiritual practices, activities or festivities
(1) not at all (2) a little (3) more or less (4) a lot (5) very much

75. I set up a place of prayer in my home
(1) not at all (2) a little (3) more or less (4) a lot (5) very much

76. I tried to deal with my feelings without asking for God's help
(1) not at all (2) a little (3) more or less (4) a lot (5) very much

77. I looked for help in the holy books
(1) not at all (2) a little (3) more or less (4) a lot (5) very much

78. I wondered what I had done to make God punish me
(1) not at all (2) a little (3) more or less (4) a lot (5) a lot

79. I tried to change my life path and follow a new one - God's way
(1) not at all (2) a little (3) more or less (4) a lot (5) a lot

80. I tried to talk to my higher self
(1) not at all (2) a little (3) more or less (4) a lot (5) very much

81. I turned to spirituality
(1) not at all (2) a little (3) more or less (4) a lot (5) a lot

82. I sought God's help to get rid of my bad/negative feelings
(1) not at all (2) a little (3) more or less (4) a lot (5) a lot

83. I blamed God for the situation, for letting it happen
(1) not at all (2) a little (3) more or less (4) a lot (5) a lot

84. I wondered if God really cared
(1) not at all (2) a little (3) more or less (4) a lot (5) very much

85. I prayed individually and did what I identified with most spiritually
(1) not at all (2) a little (3) more or less (4) a lot (5) a lot

86. I wondered if I wasn't going against God's laws and tried to change my attitude
(1) not at all (2) a little (3) more or less (4) a lot (5) a lot

87. I sought a house of God
1)) not at all (2) a little (3) more or less (4) a lot (5) a lot

THANKS FOR TAKING PART!

ANNEX 2- GENERAL QUESTIONNAIRE

(Demographic, socio-economic, religious and health data)
1) DATE: *|______/2010* **2) AGE 3) SEX:** 1 ()M 2 ()F

4) What is your level of education?
1 () incomplete primary education (up to grade level); 5 () incomplete higher education;
2 ()   completed primary school;6 () completed higher education;
3 ()   incomplete secondary education; 7 () incomplete postgraduate degree;
4 ()   completed secondary education; 8 () completed   postgraduate   studies.

5) Approximately what is your family's monthly income?
1 ()   1 minimum wage4 () between 5 and 10 minimum wages
2 ()   2 to 3 minimum wages5 () more than 10 minimum wages
3 ()   up to 5 minimum wages6 () more than 20 minimum wages

6) What is your marital status?
1 ( ) Single 2 ( ) Married 3 ( ) Divorced 4 ( ) Widowed 5 ( ) Other. Which?

**7) For you ,   what   is
God?** ____

8) Do you believe in God (power, spirit, intelligence or superior force, etc)?
1 () Yes 2 () No

9) If yes, for how long?
1 () I've always believed3   () 5 years ago
2 () for 1 year4   () for 10 years
5 () for more than 10 years

10) With regard to your religion/doctrine/sect/belief, do you consider yourself...
1 () Atheist (doesn't believe in God)
2 ( ) No religion, but spiritualised (believes in God, but doesn't belong to any religion)
3 () Catholic6   () Spiritualist9   () Jewish
4 () Protestant7   () Buddhist10   () Muslim 5 () Evangelical 8 (
) Umbandist 11 () Other. Please specify:

11) Have you ever changed your religion/doctrine/belief throughout your life?
1 () No 2 () Yes, I changed to

**12) How important has religion/spirituality been in dealing with the current
stressors in your life?**
1 () Not important3   () Relatively important
2 () Somewhat important4   () Important
5 () Very important

**13)   How often do you go to church/temple/centre/yard/synagogue or any other
meetings of a religious nature?**
1 () Never5   () Twice a month
2 () Rarely6   () Once a week
3 () Once a year7   () More than once a week.
How many?___________
4 () Once a month 8 () Once a day

**14) How much time do you devote to private religious activities, such as prayer,
meditation or studying holy books (like the Bible, Talmud, Koran, etc.) or other
religious books?**
1 () Never5   ()   Once a week
2 () Rarely6   ()   Two to three times a week
3 () Once a   year7   ()   Once a day
4 () Once a   month8   ()   More than once a day

15) Regardless of whether or not you attend religious meetings, how important is religion to you?
1 () Not important3   () Relatively important
2 () Somewhat important4   () Important
5 () Very important

16) How much has religion/spirituality helped you manage or cope with the stressful situations you've experienced?
1 () It hasn't helped3   () It has helped more or less.
2 () It has helped little4   () It has helped.
5 () It has helped a lot

Think about yourself, how you have changed as a result of the stressful event(s) you have experienced and answer how much you agree with the following sentences:

17) - I have grown spiritually.
1 () I haven't grown.   3 () I've grown more or less.
2 () I've grown a bit.   4 () I've grown.
5 () I've grown a lot.

18) - I have grown with God.
1 () I haven't grown.   3 () I've grown more or less.
2 () I've grown a bit.   4 () I've grown.
5 () I've grown a lot.

19) - I have grown up with my religious institution (my church, temple, centre, quarry, synagogue, mosque, among others)
1 () I haven't grown.   3 () I've grown more or less.
2 () I've grown a bit.   4 () I've grown.
5 () I've grown a lot.

Considering your body and mind, answer the questions below:

20) - How do you rate your health? (Describe or explain in your own words).

21) - How would you rate your health?
1 () Very bad2   () Weak 3 () Neither bad nor good
4 () Good. 5 () Very good.

22 - Do you consider yourself...
1 () Healthy2   () Sick.

23 - Do you have any health problems?
1- () No 2- () Yes, I have

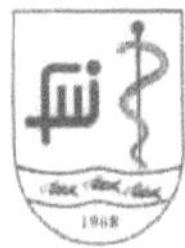

FACULDADE DE MEDICINA DE JUNDIAÍ

Autarquia Municipal criada por Lei Municipal Nº 1506 de 12 de março de 1966 - C.N.P.J Nº 50.955.266/0001-09
Reconhecimento Federal Decreto Nº 71656 de 04/01/1973

R. Francisco Telles, 250 - CEP: 13.202-550 - Cx. Postal: 1295
Fone/Fax: (11) 4587-1095 - Jundiaí-SP - site: www.fmj.br - e-mail: fmj@fmj.br

COMITÊ DE ÉTICA EM PESQUISA

Jundiaí, 2 de junho de 2010

Ilustríssima Senhora
ANA CLÁUDIA GIESBRECHT PUGGINA

Ref.: Aprovação a Projeto de Pesquisa.

Título: "Coping Religioso-Espiritual dos Familiares de Pacientes Internados em Unidade de Terapia Intensiva".

Prezada Pesquisadora:

O Comitê de Ética em Pesquisa – CEP desta Faculdade, em reunião no dia 2 de junho de 2010, no cumprimento de suas atribuições e após revisão ao seu protocolo de pesquisa em epígrafe, emitiu parecer APROVANDO os seguintes documentos:

» Versão nº 1 do Protocolo de Pesquisa original, de março de 2010.
» Versão nº 2 do Termo de Consentimento Livre e Esclarecido, de maio de 2010.

Lembramos a V.Sa. que é necessário enviar a este CEP relatórios semestrais e relatório de eventos adversos, caso estes venham a ocorrer, assim como relatório final com os resultados da pesquisa, para finalização do processo. Quaisquer dúvidas estamos à disposição.

Atenciosamente,

Prof. Dr. Rogério Bonassi Machado
Coordenador do Comitê de Ética em Pesquisa

APPENDIX 1 - INFORMED CONSENT FORM FOR FAMILY MEMBERS

Research title: Religious-Spiritual Coping of Family Members of Patients in an Intensive Care Unit.
Researcher: Academic Letícia Preti Schleder
Supervisor: Prof. Ms Ana Cláudia Giesbrecht Puggina

You are being invited to take part in a research study. Your participation is completely voluntary. Before deciding whether to take part, it is important that you understand what will be carried out and what the research will involve. Please read the following information and ask if anything is unclear or if you would like more information.

This study aims to assess their religious and spiritual coping with the stress of hospitalisation.

Data collection will be carried out in the waiting room of the KICUs, initially with a questionnaire to characterise the research subjects, containing 23 questions, and then the *Religious-Spiritual Coping Scale*, which contains a total of 87 items.

The data collection time will be approximately 40 minutes, and the privacy of the participants' data will be maintained. If you wish, you can leave the study, as there will be no repression of any kind. The results of the study will be used exclusively for scientific purposes.

I declare that I have been given all the information about this study, and I hereby undertake to take part in the research. Should there be any further questions on this subject, I can contact the student researcher Letícia Preti Schleder via e-mail: ticiapreti@hotmail.com or mobile: (11)7193- 9949.

I am aware that if I have any questions or feel harmed, I can contact the researcher responsible, or the Research Ethics Committee of the Jundiaí Medical School, located at Rua Francisco Telles, 250, Vila Arens, Jundiaí, CEP:13202-550, telephone (11)4587-1095 I,.., bearer of the R.G .... I have been informed of the objectives of the above research in a clear and detailed manner. The researcher Letícia Preti Schleder has assured me that all the data from this research will be used for scientific purposes only.

I declare that I have received a copy of this Consent Form,

Jundiaí, 2010.

_______________________________   _______________________________
Academic Leticia Preti Schleder   Participant's signature
      Researcher

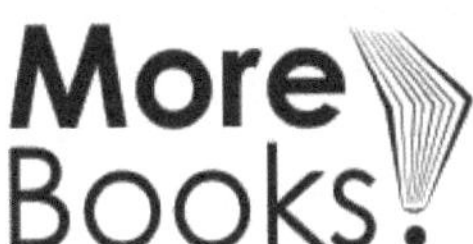

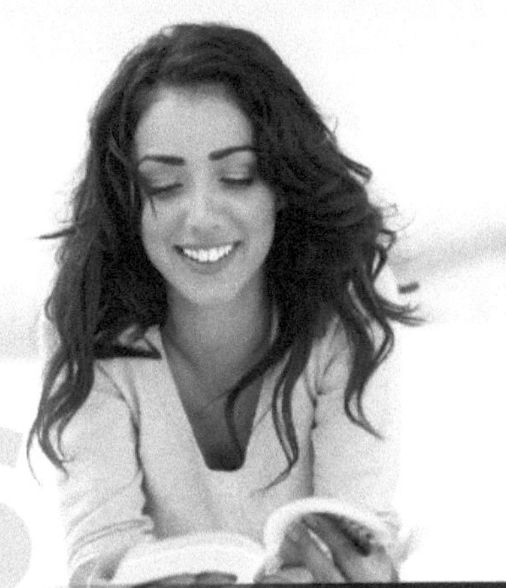

I want morebooks!

Buy your books fast and straightforward online - at one of world's fastest growing online book stores! Environmentally sound due to Print-on-Demand technologies.

Buy your books online at
www.morebooks.shop

Kaufen Sie Ihre Bücher schnell und unkompliziert online – auf einer der am schnellsten wachsenden Buchhandelsplattformen weltweit! Dank Print-On-Demand umwelt- und ressourcenschonend produzi ert.

Bücher schneller online kaufen
www.morebooks.shop

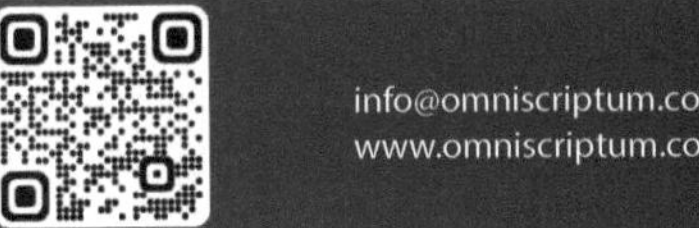

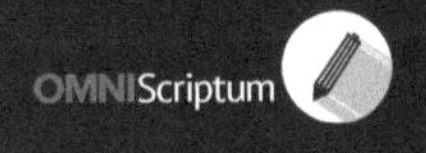

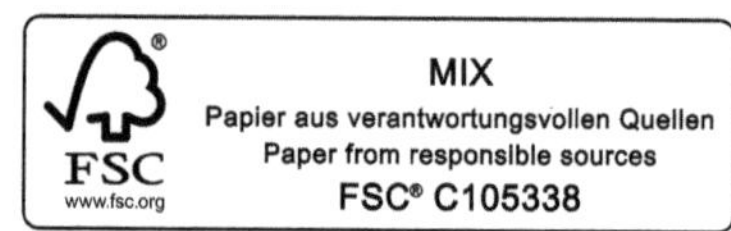

Printed by Books on Demand GmbH, Norderstedt / Germany